Mental Health Resilience

Mental Health Resilience

The Social Context of Coping with Mental Illness

ABIGAIL GOSSELIN

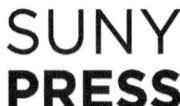

Published by State University of New York Press, Albany

© 2024 State University of New York

All rights reserved

Printed in the United States of America

No part of this book may be used or reproduced in any manner whatsoever without written permission. No part of this book may be stored in a retrieval system or transmitted in any form or by any means including electronic, electrostatic, magnetic tape, mechanical, photocopying, recording, or otherwise without the prior permission in writing of the publisher.

For information, contact State University of New York Press, Albany, NY
www.sunypress.edu

Library of Congress Cataloging-in-Publication Data

Name: Gosselin, Abigail, 1977- author.
Title: Mental health resilience : the social context of coping with mental illness / Abigail Gosselin.
Description: Albany : State University of New York Press, [2024] | Includes bibliographical references and index.
Identifiers: LCCN 2023042518 | ISBN 9781438497808 (hardcover : alk. paper) | ISBN 9781438497822 (ebook) | ISBN 9781438497815 (pbk. : alk. paper)
Subjects: LCSH: Mental illness—Social aspects. | Mentally ill—Services for. | Mentally ill—Social conditions. | Mental health services.
Classification: LCC RC455 .G653 2024 | DDC 362.2—dc23/eng/20240209
LC record available at https://lccn.loc.gov/2023042518

10 9 8 7 6 5 4 3 2 1

To Derrick

Contents

Acknowledgments		ix
Introduction		1
Chapter 1	Enabling Mental Health Resilience	11
Chapter 2	Vulnerabilities of Mental Illness	39
Chapter 3	Inner Resources	71
Chapter 4	Social Support	99
Chapter 5	Resources for Meeting People's Needs	129
Chapter 6	Resources for Social Justice	155
Chapter 7	Opportunities for Meaning	183
Conclusion		209
Notes		215
Bibliography		241
Index		255

Acknowledgments

Thank you to my colleagues at Regis University, my scholarly home for over a decade, and particularly to my department members: Karen Adkins, Ron DiSanto, Anandita Mukherji, Jason Taylor, Becky Vartabedian, and Ted Zenzinger. A special thank you goes to Ted, who read an early draft of the manuscript and helped me reconceptualize and restructure it to make it a better book. In addition, I am grateful to three anonymous reviewers whose insightful comments helped improve the book.

I greatly appreciate the love and support that my parents, Deb and Marc Gosselin, and my sister and her partner, Joanne Gosselin and Jason Carter, have given me over the years. Moreover, the love and support of my husband, Derrick Belanger, and my children, Rhea and Phoebe Belanger, have been instrumental in my success. Thank you for always being there for me. And thank you for believing in me.

Introduction

At the end of her provocative memoir about her experiences with schizophrenia, law professor Elyn Saks expresses the value of a good life for everyone, including those with mental illness: "What I rather wish to say is that the humanity we all share is more important than the mental illness we may not. With proper treatment, someone who is mentally ill can lead a full and rich life. What makes life wonderful—good friends, a satisfying job, loving relationships—is just as valuable for those of us who struggle with schizophrenia as for anyone else."[1] Even while struggling with illness, people can acquire the components of a good life, including supportive friends, care from loved ones, and a job or other activity that provides meaning. In order to achieve these aspects of a good life, however, they must learn how to cope successfully with their illness. And in order to cope, they must develop some resilience.

Ken Steele, who also recovered from schizophrenia, conveys his hope for the future at the end of his memoir, *The Day the Voices Stopped*. He looks forward to a time when people with mental illness will no longer live secluded from society but rather be integrated into it, living the kinds of lives that those without mental illness are capable of living: "I have a vision that goes like this: In this new century [the twenty-first century], mentally ill people will have the science, the organized voting strength, and the means to leave our ghettos of isolation behind us. We will finally join with the mainstream community, where we'll be able to live as independent individuals and not as a group of people who are known and feared by the names of our illness."[2] In his vision, Steele imagines that mental illness will no longer dominate a person's life and the way they are seen by society; instead, a person will be able to manage their illness and not be defined by it.

In order for a person to avoid having illness control their life and to be able to live a life of meaning despite having illness—and thus, in a certain sense, to be able to engage in recovery—they must have the resources, support, and opportunities that enable them to manage their illness and grow from it rather than be diminished by it. Living a life beyond illness requires having the resilience to cope with struggles and to adapt to changing and challenging circumstances, a resilience that can only be attained through the support of individuals and institutions that can provide the resources and opportunities needed to cope. Steele's hope for the future is attainable—if society supports those with mental illness by providing them with the tools they need.

Resilience is the capacity to cope with difficult circumstances by changing the situation or—when one lacks the power to change one's situation—by changing oneself to adapt. With resilience, people can deal with adversity successfully, in a way that allows them to flourish as human beings. Resilience is a necessary component of recovery from mental illness, for people can learn to cope with their illness, even if they cannot control the fact that they have illness or how it manifests, when they have the tools that enable them to cope. As this book argues, society plays an important role in creating the conditions that allow people to be resilient, making it possible for people with mental illness to cope with their illness successfully. With adequate support, resources, and opportunities, individuals and institutions in society can provide what is needed so that people with mental illness have the resilience to be able to recover.

I started thinking about resilience after my recovery from psychosis in the early 2020s. Having been diagnosed with bipolar I disorder when I was twenty-five years old, I cycled through manic, depressive, and mixed episodes (interspersed with periods of feeling "normal") for over a dozen years. Then, in 2017, I had a psychotic break and struggled with psychosis for much of the next two years, sometimes also depressed and suicidal and sometimes not. When I was very depressed and psychotic in April 2018, I was hospitalized for a week; after that, I spent months in an intensive outpatient program in between teaching my classes.[3]

Over the course of these two years of being sick with psychosis and depression, I made several medication changes as my psychiatrist tried to stabilize me with various antipsychotic, antidepressant, and antianxiety medications. When I reached a sufficient dose of mirtazapine in January 2019, the suicidal thoughts and depression finally went away. It wasn't until I was on a relatively high dose of ziprasidone and a small dose of risperidone, beginning in July 2019, that the psychosis finally receded.

Recovery did not happen immediately; it took me many months of working hard after beginning the risperidone to be able to recover. Although the risperidone eliminated the strange experiences I had been having—what are chalked up as hallucinations and delusions—it did not by itself make me better. I had learned all kinds of harmful habits of thought and feeling, and I had developed a dependency on my husband and a sense of helplessness and lack of autonomy and agency. Now in recovery, I had to relearn how to make decisions for myself and how to act in the world and interact with others appropriately. After two years of feeling generally incompetent, I had to relearn how to be competent at many activities in my life, and I had to develop the confidence and trust in myself that I could handle whatever came my way. After about a year of no longer being psychotic, I finally started to feel "normal" and started to learn to trust myself to be able to act in the world in the right sorts of ways.

As I continued my recovery, I wondered what it was that enabled me to recover besides being on the right medication. What attitudes did I have to have to be able to try new treatments, to do what my psychiatrist and therapist suggested, and to participate consistently in my recovery? What skills did I learn that were useful, and what virtues did I develop in working on my recovery? What inner resources was I able to draw upon and what external resources did I need to rely upon to make recovery possible? How did having more privilege than the average person with severe mental illness help me to recover more easily? In short, I wondered what made me resilient during this time of recovery.

During the two years that I was sick, every step forward in my healing (for example, attending therapy and psychiatrist appointments, trying to do what my doctor and therapist suggested) was accompanied by a step back and a return of the psychosis and/or suicidal thoughts. During this time, I could not sustain positive change. While I was sick, recovery had seemed impossible, which made me feel like I was incapable of getting better. What, besides medication, made it different this time? What enabled me to get better after two years of feeling so stuck?

Resilience is the process of being able to deal with adversity by learning how to manage difficult situations, and oneself, so that one is not torn apart by the experience of difficulty. When I was sick, psychosis severed me by destroying my sense of self, agency, autonomy, and identity. At times, I welcomed the strange experiences I was having and let the psychosis do what it would to me. At other times, when I was in sufficient despair, I tried taking steps to manage the psychosis, such as trying new medications and trying different therapeutic techniques my therapist recommended. But I could never manage it sufficiently to not be undone by it. The psychosis always came back, with full force, as if I hadn't done anything to try to mitigate it. Until it didn't.

After trying the risperidone, and practicing many techniques my therapist taught me, I was finally able to manage the psychosis—and myself—so that the psychosis no longer undid me. Remnants of psychosis remained, but I was able to control them. With intensive outpatient therapy and weekly sessions with my talk therapist, I had changed enough of my self—improving my agency and autonomy, increasing my capabilities and competence in many things, getting better at accepting what I couldn't control, and taking responsibility for what I could—that I could deal with the difficulties of psychosis itself and the effects it had had on me for those years. I had changed myself, and I was able to manage my circumstances better so psychosis no longer locked me in its grip. And I wondered: How did I eventually become resilient enough to be able to deal with psychosis and its aftermath? How was I finally able to change after so many times of trying?

My heroes have always been the people who face significant adversity—particularly the inner demons of various forms of psychological torment—and are compromised by that adversity, yet somehow manage to continue to fight it. They are the people who, no matter how many times adversity knocks them down, and no matter how many times they have to try again, reengage the fight as many times as it takes. They don't give up, not for good. They might give up temporarily—inner demons tend to make us give up on ourselves at some points—but they somehow manage to reengage. The perseverance involved with fighting adversity is what I admire most in people. People who are resilient have this perseverance: they continue to reengage, trying to manage their adversity, no matter how many times and how badly it knocks them down.

The particular people whom I have admired have changed over time. When I was younger, and my manic and depressive states were overwhelming, I admired other bipolar individuals and fixated on Scott Weiland, who was the lead singer for the 1990s band Stone Temple Pilots. I interpreted all of his songs as being about being knocked down and getting back up to fight, and I was deeply inspired by what I saw as his resilience, his perseverance in not ultimately giving up. Over the years, I developed fantastical beliefs tying my own fate to his, so that when he ultimately died of a drug overdose, I thought it was a premonition of my own demise. Antipsychotic medication has released me from these delusions so that I no longer connect my fate to his. Rather, I am sorry that he ultimately lost the fight. I am also grateful for, and inspired by, all the fighting he did along the way.

Today my heroes tend to be people who have suffered from psychosis and have learned how to live successful lives on their own terms, managing their illness so it does not rule their lives. I am especially inspired by people like Steele and Saks, both of whom have overcome significant difficulties related to their experiences with psychosis in order to live meaningful and purposive lives. This book borrows from their stories to offer a more complete and humanistic account of the kind of resilience necessary to address mental illness. There is much we can learn from the experiences of others. In my analysis, I draw upon the experience of Steele and Saks to explore what resilience is in the context of recovery from mental illness and what it requires. I summarize aspects of these individuals' stories and reflect on the significance of their experiences throughout this book.

One of the major themes that arises from looking at these two individuals' stories is that social and institutional support is necessary for people to be able to cope with mental illness, but that social and institutional support, in order to be efficacious, must be just. As we shall see, Saks believed that she could overcome her mental illness on her own if she only tried hard enough, but she learned through many setbacks that she could not do this alone; she needed social and institutional help. It was necessary for institutions and individuals to provide the support, resources, and opportunities required for resilience. At the same time, supplying aid and support is not sufficient; as we shall see from Steele's story, resources, support, and opportunities need to be provided in just ways in order for people to be able to access and use them efficaciously. Steele was victim to many different kinds of structural injustices in our society and was only able to access the resources, support, and opportunities he needed when the systems that he was working within were structured more justly. Being able to cope with mental illness requires social and institutional support, which must be given in a context of social justice.

Being beaten down by illness and then finding ways to manage it without losing one's agency, autonomy, and identity is something that many people with mental illness experience in the process of recovery. Mental illness makes people vulnerable to specific kinds of harms, some direct and others indirect, which can cause a person to lose functioning, agency, and autonomy. Mental illness interferes with people's basic need for mental health, sometimes making it difficult for a person to go on living as a human being. When people find ways to manage their mental health challenges, they are often able to recover from mental illness, not in the sense that mental illness disappears—for some people, it is never eliminated—but in the sense that it no longer has to dominate a person's life.

Recovery from mental illness can be understood as finding a way to go on living and having a rich, full life despite having mental illness. It involves figuring out how to live the kind of life a person wishes to live, given the constraints they have. Recovery is a nonlinear journey that can involve various obstacles and setbacks, not necessarily progressing toward a continuously better end, but progressing nevertheless toward the ends a person desires at a given time, based on where they are at that time. While vulnerabilities can create major constraints that people have to deal with and work around, recovery provides them with the openings and options that allow them possibilities in going forth.

Recovery requires resilience, because it requires that people learn how to cope with their illness so that they control it rather than the other way around, and how to direct themselves in ways that allow them to cope. When a person finds a way to manage their mental illness, they are able to mitigate the losses mental illness tends to produce and sometimes even grow from their experiences of adversity, making it easier for a person to go on living, and even to flourish, despite having illness. Overcoming mental illness is not always possible; sometimes people live with illness for long periods, even their whole adult lives. Yet they can still be in recovery from mental illness when they are able to live meaningful lives despite their illness.

Understanding the types of vulnerability mental illness produces and the kind of resilience needed to address it involves, for me (as a philosopher), philosophical analyses of resilience, vulnerability, responsibility, internal and external resources, social support, and meaning. While resilience is addressed extensively in some fields, including psychology, ecology, engineering, and crisis management, it has not been studied to the same degree in philosophy. A philosophical account of resilience in the context of mental illness requires assessment of the concept of resilience; analysis of the concept of vulnerability to better understand the nature of harm to which mental illness subjects people; delineation of social support; analysis of responsibility for getting basic needs met and for creating structural justice; examination of meaning; and analysis of necessary components of resilience, including internal and external resources, support, and opportunities.

This book begins with an assessment of the concept of resilience, arguing that we should understand resilience not as "bouncing back" from adversity but rather as having the capacity to mobilize adequate resources, support, and opportunities effectively to deal with adversity in a way that enables a person to flourish as a human being by increasing their core capacities of agency, autonomy, and meaning-making. Resilience is traditionally thought of as the responsibility of the individuals coping with adversity to cope on their own, but in fact resilience typically has a social context where people learn how to be resilient from others and where they acquire the tools necessary for resilience from society. Resilience is thus the responsibility of all individuals and institutions within a society; individuals and institutions create the conditions that enable resilience by providing people with the resources, support, and opportunities necessary for coping with mental health and other life challenges.

Chapter 2 analyzes the concept of vulnerability as it applies to mental illness, explicating the various types of vulnerabilities to which people with mental illness are subject. Mental illness makes people especially vulnerable because of the way it creates and exacerbates a wide variety of potential and actual harms, compounding a person's vulnerability. Many of the harms that people are subject to are social in nature, arising from the ways that people are situated in relation to others within their society; addressing these vulnerabilities thus requires addressing the social conditions that give rise to them.

In chapters 3–7, I examine what inner resources and external resources, support, and opportunities are required for resilience, showing how these all have a social context in that they can only be obtained through social provision and social interaction. Chapter 3 shows that people develop the inner resources that enable resilience only through social interaction and learning from others. People can cope with their circumstances only by changing them (when they have control over them) or by adjusting to them (when they do not) when they learn the requisite virtues, skills, and dispositions through social engagement.

Social interventions provide the means that enable resilience. Chapters 4–7 look at what responsibilities individuals and institutions have to provide the resources, support, and opportunities that people need to be able to cope with adversity. Social support is delineated in chapter 4, which argues that individuals have a duty to protect the vulnerable and a duty to care. Both of these duties require people to interact intentionally with those who have mental illness in ways that support them, which helps diminish their mental disorder symptoms and makes life more manageable for them.

The responsibilities of institutions to realize people's human rights and to create structural justice are analyzed in chapters 5 and 6. Chapter 5 argues that the vulnerability of individuals gives rise to the responsive state, which creates institutions specifically designed to realize people's human rights in part by meeting their basic needs. As the United Nations recognizes, individuals have a right to mental health, which must be fulfilled by institutions that have as their responsibility to meet people's mental healthcare needs by providing them with the resources and opportunities needed for resilience. Chapter 6 argues that institutions have duties of structural justice to create conditions that are just so as not to subject people to negative social factors that imperil mental health. Part of how they accomplish this is by carrying out duties to listen and to be responsive to the needs and concerns of vulnerable individuals.

Opportunities for finding and creating meaning and purpose in one's life experiences are explored in chapter 7. One of the factors that enables resilience is the ability to find and create meaning through social engagement, meaning-making, and participating in meaningful activities such as work. When people interact with others in meaningful ways, they develop support and a sense of belonging that helps them cope with difficulty. When people are able to engage in cognitive reappraisal and narrative construction, they can make sense of their experience by making it intelligible. And when people participate in meaningful activities such as work, caretaking, volunteering, making art, and being in nature, they can experience the present moment peacefully as well as develop and work toward goals that are meaningful to them. By creating meaning in their lives, vulnerable people can use this meaning and purpose to help themselves cope with difficult circumstances such as mental illness and other life challenges.

This book is primarily intended for philosophers, students, and other academics interested in the topic of resilience, as there are no book-length treatments of resilience in the field of philosophy besides anthologies, and a philosophical analysis of the concept is badly needed. However, the book is also useful for mental health professionals and the institutions they work for who want to better understand how they can support people with mental illness in their recovery; this book shows that interventions must be pluralistic and focus in part on increasing social connections, social interactions, and social relationships, as well as social provisions of resources and opportunities. In addition, the book can be used to guide policy around mental health services, as it explores the institutional responsibility that various institutions within a state government have to protect, support, and meet the needs of people with mental illness. Finally, the book may also be useful to individuals supporting people with mental illness who want a better understanding of the social context required for resilience and recovery so they can better understand the parameters of their own responsibility in offering support.

Some of my examination of what is needed for resilience applies to other contexts besides mental health. In any context, people need their basic needs to be met and to be protected from harms and injustices so that they can exercise their inner resources and mobilize the external resources, opportunities, and support necessary for resilience. Care and protection provide necessary support to people undergoing any kind of adversity. In order to face any kind of difficulty, individuals need opportunities to develop inner resources and to find meaning and purpose, which help in resilience. Thus, while my focus is on the resilience needed by people with mental illness, and the requirements that enable that resilience, some of my arguments apply more broadly to anyone facing adversity.

Resilience is a key component of recovery for many people who have mental illness, yet it is not always clear what is needed for people to be able to be resilient. This book shows that resilience has a necessarily social context in which individuals and institutions both play a role in creating the conditions that enable resilience. They do this by providing the resources, support, and opportunities that people need in order to cope with their mental health struggles. In this way, they can contribute to people's recovery from mental illness.

Chapter 1

Enabling Mental Health Resilience

Introduction

Elyn Saks and Ken Steele are heroes of mine because, despite the extreme mental health difficulties they experienced, they persevered: they faced their challenges and fought their demons. They did not always win; sometimes their psychosis and social circumstances got the best of them. But they did win sometimes. By the time they wrote their respective memoirs—Saks's *The Center Cannot Hold* and Steele's *The Day the Voices Stopped*—they had recovered enough to be able to be self-reflective about their experience. Through the process of writing their memoirs, they exercised significant agency, autonomy, and meaning-making, showing personal growth and development in their self-reflection. They were not cured, but they were in a position from which they could direct their lives as they chose, and they had achieved self-awareness and self-knowledge. They succeeded in living a good life despite having illness in part by mobilizing the support, resources, and opportunities that they had access to in order to cope with their mental health and other life challenges. In short, they demonstrated resilience.

Saks and Steele showed resilience when they were temporarily defeated by their psychosis and (in Steele's case) suicidality, yet still managed to go on. Saks demonstrates this vividly in her description of how she dealt with being psychotic for two weeks following a grade she was unhappy with. During this time, she didn't eat or shower, she muttered to herself, she shuffled around her apartment, and she spent significant time curled up in a ball on her bed. Her psychiatrist prescribed a higher dose of her antipsychotic medication, and she very reluctantly took it. She says, "Gradually, the increased dose of Navane kicked in, the demons receded, and the fog lifted. I got up off the floor, cleaned myself up, and one more time I went back out into the world and started all over again."[1] She needed the treatment prescribed to her by her mental health professional in order to be able to recover from this psychotic episode; with that help, she was able to go on. She did not remain stuck in her psychosis, as she was surely tempted; instead, she fought off the psychosis and went on with her life. This ability to go on, despite wanting to give up and succumb to one's inner demons, is resilience.

Saks worked hard at keeping her psychosis at bay. When experiencing delusions, she would tell herself to "hold it together."[2] She was extraordinary in her ability to engage in such self-talk, as many people with paranoid delusions lack enough insight into their illness to be able to recognize, assess, and respond to symptoms in this way. This positive self-talk was a way of managing her symptoms so she could do the things she wanted to do without having the psychosis overcome her.

Her determination to deal with her problems gave her the motivation and energy she needed to do so. With this determination, she could fight against her psychosis, aware that sometimes it could defeat her, but that other times she could overcome it. She states, "Every time I'd been knocked down, I'd gotten back up again. There was no reason why I couldn't keep doing it. I just had to control my mind, not vice versa, and if I was careful, I would be able to claim and fully inhabit the life I wanted."[3] By fighting against her inner demons, she could take control over her life in a context where her psychosis often seemed to control her. In this way, she could reestablish her agency and autonomy in exercising her resilience.

Steele showed similar perseverance when he fought against his voices. He says, "I worked in spite of my delusional voices and because of them: I was going to prove them wrong."[4] Although he could not control his voices and make them go away, he could defy them by acting in ways that were contrary to their dictates. For example, for a time he worked at a medical library and then at a garden in work placements given to him by the rehabilitative program that helped him, the Fountain clubhouse in New York City. It would have been easy to succumb to the voices and give up trying to live in the real world, but he was able to persevere and fight against this tendency.

While he was often overcome by his voices, living in a fantasy world they ruled, he occasionally found ways to get himself the help he needed.

Sometimes this involved voluntarily going to an emergency room to be hospitalized; later in his life, this involved finding a good therapist whom he sought out on his own. Since the therapist pushed him hard to talk about childhood trauma, he started to resist therapy, breaking several appointments he had made, and eventually he stopped seeing her in order to avoid the hard work she was pushing him to do. After he was beaten down by his illness again, however, he recognized that she had really been helping him, and he tried to see her and make amends. " 'I want to come back and continue the hard work we were doing,' I said."[5] His ability to reach out and advocate for himself through his suffering showed strength and resilience and was an exercise of autonomous agency.

For both Saks and Steele, fighting against their inner demons and dealing with their psychoses was not easy. Saks describes how exhausting it was to try to manage her psychosis and live the life she wanted to live. She says, "The constant effort to keep reality on one side and delusions on the other was exhausting, and I often felt beaten down, knowing that the schizophrenia diagnosis had ended any hope I'd had of a miracle cure or a miracle fix."[6] It would have been easier to give up and live in her delusional world, but she had enough determination to live her self-chosen life to want to fight against this.

Similarly, Steele describes the agony and despair of trying and not succeeding. During a time when he was living in a halfway house and working at jobs the rehabilitative program helped set him up with, he was trying hard to make a living and do things that were meaningful to him. But after a setback, when the baby of a nurse he cared about died, he blamed himself for the tragedy and his voices came roaring back. (Elsewhere he describes how being psychotic made him feel like he was the center of the universe, that everything happened because of him.[7]) He says, "It was one of the worst psychotic storms of my life. I was bombarded by the voices and overcome by self-loathing. Here I'd been trying so hard to achieve some kind of useful life, but every attempt resulted in disaster and I was back where I started: damned. I *had* to be damned to hell, just as my grandmother had prophesied when I told her about my voices. Damned to wander the world a loner."[8]

In other places, he mentions a strong tendency to feel defeated by his voices. He says, "No matter what advances I fought long and hard to make, the ever-present voices had the power to reverse my efforts."[9] Even though he tried to fight the voices, he often didn't win. Frequently, the voices overpowered him and dictated what he did and how he saw and interacted with the world. Yet, despite this powerful feeling of defeat, he did not, in the end, give up. He might go through bad periods, but he also went through good periods where he sought out help, worked, lived in halfway houses, had friends, and managed his illness. He successfully persevered through the bad periods, showing resilience in his ability to fight against his condition and deal with his challenges.

As we see from Steele's and Saks's stories, one characteristic that is often seen as essential to coping with mental illness and making a life of meaning for oneself is having resilience. Resilience means, roughly, overcoming adversity, and it involves drawing upon a variety of inner resources as well as external resources to be able to face challenges and deal with them in constructive ways. People who have mental illness and who are resilient are able to deal with their mental illness symptoms and the social, psychological, and physical effects of being mentally ill more effectively than those who are not resilient. Resilience aids in recovery from mental illness because it allows people to cope with their mental illness in ways that do not exacerbate the illness, and it allows people to respond to life stressors in ways that do not contribute to further mental illness. With resilience, people who have mental illness can find a way to live with their illness without letting it rule their life.

Resilience is thus considered an important aspect of recovery from mental illness. But what constitutes resilience is open to debate, as theorists define resilience in different ways. While resilience is intended to be a helpful construct, enabling a person to live a better life despite difficulties, some conceptions of resilience are actually problematic, hurting a person as much as helping them. In this chapter I examine different definitions of resilience and determine that a good way to understand it is maintaining integrity as a human being—and maintaining or developing capacities of agency, autonomy, and meaning-making—while changing or adapting to difficult circumstances. Resilience thus involves transformation of one's situation or oneself as a way of coping.

Next, I consider objections to traditional understandings of resilience, focusing especially on the way it tends to be individualistic, locating control and responsibility in the individual facing adversity rather than in social institutions that may have helped create the adversity or that have as their role to aid people experiencing adversity. This leads me to revise my definition of resilience as involving the capacity to mobilize adequate resources, support, and opportunities effectively to deal with challenges in a manner that enables a person to exercise their basic human capacities so that they can function in various areas of their life and flourish as a human being. Resources, support, and opportunities include both those that come from within a person, which are developed in a relational context through social interactions and social relationships with others, and those that are external to a person, which are provided through social institutions and practices. Resilience is only effective in a social context that supports the person experiencing challenges and gives them the tools to be able to address challenges.

Let us start with the idea of resilience as overcoming adversity and examine different definitions to see what this can mean.

Definitions of Resilience

Resilience is a broad concept used in many different fields, including psychology, engineering, crisis management, and ecology. In general, it means coping with difficulties, but what it means to "cope" differs in various understandings of the term. Here I examine some of the predominant ways resilience is discussed in the relevant literatures, focusing ultimately on the psychological context that is relevant for thinking about resilience in the face of mental illness.

Returning to or Reaching a Baseline, or Achieving Equilibrium

In some traditional understandings of resilience, it is thought to involve overcoming adversity by returning to some sort of a baseline, either a return to a previous state that one was in before encountering the adversity, or a new state involving reaching some goal that has been set out. The idea of "bouncing back" from adversity, for example, suggests returning to one's original state or coming to a newer and better state.[10] The idea of achieving equilibrium is another way to understand this return to an original state or development of a new and better state. Some accounts of resilience involve achieving an equilibrium, either the old system of stability one has before adversity, or a new system of balance that has changed in response to adversity.[11] In either case, a baseline is established that a system or person tries to attain for the sake of achieving balance, stability, or homeostasis.

Theorists today tend to reject the idea of resilience as returning to a previous state or system of equilibrium, recognizing that this is not always attainable after experiencing adversity or significant change. Mianna Lotz notes that adversity can permanently transform a person in such a way that returning to a pre-adversity level of functioning may not be possible.[12] Moreover, even if it is attainable, returning to a previous state or system of equilibrium is not always desirable. Sometimes experiencing adversity sheds light on shortcomings that a person or system has that can—and ought to—be remedied while coping with difficulties. It may be desirable to change in order to better deal with future adversity, or in order simply to function in a more positive way.

Resilience as reaching a goal state is also problematic, because the goals one sets for what this baseline should look like may not reflect what is actually attainable. Moreover, a system or person may achieve growth and development by dealing with adversity that go beyond what any goal baseline can account for. Baselines in general are not helpful for thinking about resilience because they ignore some of the most important aspects of resilience. A person or system may achieve a better state than the state they were in before adversity, but what makes them resilient is not the achievement of this state but rather the process of change they underwent in approaching this state.

Achieving a new equilibrium, one which may be unforeseen and unable to plan for, may occur in relation to dealing with difficulty, but it is not clear if equilibrium or stability is always desirable. Sometimes the best way to deal with significant change is to be open to further significant changes and to change oneself continuously in response. Achieving equilibrium often involves looking backward at the stability a person or system experienced before adversity, at least for the sake of comparison, but resilience often involves looking and pushing forward, too, which psychologists describe as sustainability. Sustainability involves learning, growing, planning, adopting ends, and figuring out ways to achieve those ends.[13] Sustainability does not always lead to stability and equilibrium, and it is not clear that it needs to.

Maintaining Identity

One component that is often identified as important to resilience is maintaining identity or integrity. In the context of system resilience, Charles Redman defines resilience as "the capacity of a system to experience shocks while retaining function, structure, feedback capabilities, and therefore identity."[14] Brian Walker and David Salt similarly describe resilience as "the capacity of a system to absorb disturbance and reorganize so as to retain essentially the same function, structure, and feedbacks—to have the same identity," and "the ability to cope with shocks and keep functioning in much the same kind of way."[15]

Here significant change is understood as shocks or disturbances, something that seriously shakes up the system. Coping with shocks can be understood as the system keeping its identity by holding on to some of its core features, including its function, its structure, and its feedback capabilities, despite undergoing radical change. Some stability is maintained through and despite change when certain key aspects of a system are able to remain the same through the change.

While Redman and Walker and Salt focus on the resilience of systems, William Throop focuses on the resilience of individuals, offering a similar definition. For him, resilience involves "enabling something to bounce back from adversity while retaining function and identity."[16] Here resilience is about "bouncing back" from difficulties, which we might understand as overcoming difficulties without undergoing significant harm. What is key here is the idea of retaining function and identity through difficulties. Here, a person is resilient when they can endure adversity without losing function or identity. I address the idea of function later; here we are looking at the role of identity. Whether identity is to be understood as personal identity or the identity of oneself as a human being is unclear.

In the context of systems, the question arises as to how much change a system can endure without changing its identity. What if something interacts with a system to change its function or structure—how much of this change can occur while retaining identity, and at what threshold does the amount of change make the system change its identity? For example, a wildfire can damage an ecosystem significantly, and it can be difficult to see to what extent the ecosystem can retain its identity given the damage that occurs and to what extent it changes in a substantial way. Probably the answer about how much change a system can endure while retaining its identity will be different for different systems, as some understanding of the particular system's identity is necessary to see how elastic it is.

A similar question arises in the context of persons. How much change can a person endure without changing their identity? If we are talking about personal identity, a person's personal identity—at least, the character and personality aspects of their identity[17]—can change quite a bit in reaction to changes they undergo, yet it is not necessarily problematic to change one's personal identity. Our personal identities change all the time in response to our social and physical environments, and this is just normal. Resilience doesn't have to require us to keep our personal identities the same. This would ignore the natural dynamic nature of how we constitute ourselves in relation to our environments. Moreover, how much change a person undergoes in their personal identity seems irrelevant to how successfully they are able to deal with obstacles. Perhaps dealing with obstacles *requires* a person to change, in order to have the resources to be able to do so. Such a change would seem to be positive, something one would want to attain, not something one would want to avoid. Maintaining one's personal identity does not seem important or even relevant to resilience.

Perhaps the identity that is relevant is one's identity *as a human being*, and being human is what must not change in order for a person to be resilient. But people do undergo significant changes in some of the core aspects of what it is to be human—including their agency (ability to act on choices, based on reasons), autonomy (ability to set ends for oneself, including determining what is of value and setting goals), and meaning-making capacity (ability to assign significance, purpose, and meaning to events, experiences, objects, or people)—and yet retain the identity of being human, even if their ability to experience, exercise, and express their human capacities then becomes limited. They do not lose their humanity simply because they experience constraints on these capacities. Maintaining one's identity as human is important, but significant changes that a person can undergo do not undermine their identity as a human being, even if these changes make expressing that identity challenging. A person maintains their identity as a human being even when faced with significant difficulties and even when they react badly to those difficulties. Maintaining one's identity as a human being does not seem relevant to resilience of a person.

Since neither personal identity nor identity as a human being seems relevant to the resilience of a person, identity is not a useful concept for understanding resilience, at least in a mental health context.

Maintaining Core Function

One component of resilience that is often identified as significant is maintaining core function. Zolli and Healy define resilience as "the capacity of a system, enterprise, or a person to maintain its core purpose and integrity in the face of dramatically changed circumstances"[18] or "the ability to adapt to changed circumstances while fulfilling one's core purpose."[19] Here I'm going to focus on the core purpose aspect of this definition and address the integrity aspect later. Drawing on Zolli and Healy's account, Kelly Parker defines resilience as "the capacity to achieve one's 'core purpose' in the face of obstacles."[20] As Parker notes, on this definition resilience requires ascertaining what the core purpose of a system or person is.[21]

It is unclear whether, in the context of the person, the core purpose refers to an individual's unique sense of purpose and meaning, which they define for themselves, or the purpose of being human. Both can be relevant. One characteristic of being human is the capacity for meaning-making, and many individuals make sense of their lives by discerning purpose and meaning, seeing their experience as intelligible, and directing their lives in a way that allows them to achieve the purpose they seek and enact the meaning they perceive. Through this meaning-making, people exercise both epistemic and moral agency—the capacity to act as a knower and as a moral agent or doer—as well as autonomy—the capacity to choose the good for oneself.

Individual meaning-making is recognized by some theorists as an important part of psychological resilience. In a psychological context, John D. Mayer and Michael A. Faber understand resilience as "people's ability to cope with and find meaning in such stressful life events, in which individuals must respond with healthy individual functioning and supportive social relationships."[22] Kim Lützén and Béatrice Ewalds-Kvist associate resilience with finding meaning in all circumstances.[23] For these theorists, resilience involves making meaning out of what life has handed a person: finding meaning in the stressful events as a way of coping with them. For example, when a person is able to see what skills they have acquired as a result of dealing with stressful situations, or when a person is able to appreciate relationships that they have developed through the process of dealing with stressful situations, they can find meaning and purpose in these situations. Finding or making meaning is an individual activity that will be different for every person; this kind of meaning or purpose is subjective, up to the individual and from the individual's own perspective.

People do not need to have a subjective core purpose that they have defined for themselves in order to be able to participate in meaning-making. Individuals can find meaning in experiences, activities, and events that make sense to them in their context but do not refer to any overarching core purpose of their life. For example, a person may find playing frisbee meaningful in the sense that it is an enjoyable pastime that utilizes some of their spatial skills and hand-eye coordination, but playing frisbee may not relate to any overarching core purpose a person has, unless one of their purposes is something general like participating in activities one finds enjoyable, or exercising various skills and capacities one has. People do not need to have an overarching core purpose in their life that they can identify in order to find experiences, activities, and events meaningful.

Meaning-making should be understood as a process through which one exercises cognitive and epistemic capacities, along with autonomy and agency; it is the process of participating in meaning-making that is part of a person's core purpose, not the identification of an overarching purpose with which everything meaningful has to connect. Meaning-making should thus be understood not as subjectively determining a core purpose for oneself but rather as a process of being able to find meaning in activities, events, and experiences based on other things that are meaningful in a person's life. The core function of a person, therefore, should be understood as concerning not only subjective meaning-making but also more generally as capacities that characteristically make a person human, including agency and autonomy. Resilience understood in terms of core function is the capacity of a person to maintain their agency, autonomy, and capacity for meaning-making—and thus their integrity as a human being—in light of significant change.

This is in line with the view of individual resilience given by Alex J. Zautra, John Stuart Hall, and Kate E. Murray, as "the amount of stress that a person can endure without a fundamental change in capacity to pursue aims that give life meaning."[24] Here again, meaning-making ("giving life meaning"), autonomy (having aims), and agency ("*pursuing* aims") are seen as the core functions of a human being. Resilience involves maintaining one's integrity as a human being by maintaining the capacity to make meaning, the capacity to determine what aims are worthwhile (autonomy), and the capacity to pursue the aims one has chosen (agency).

MAINTAINING FUNCTIONING

In the psychological literature, there is another way of understanding what it is to maintain function, not in terms of core function—either individual meaning and purpose, or the core function of being human—but rather in terms of functioning in life domains. William Throop understands resilience in a psychological context as "the ability to adapt to external changes and to handle stressors without losing functioning."[25] This functioning may include physical, mental, psychological, and social functioning, as well as functioning in various life domains such as work, school, social relationships, leisure activities, and civic engagement, even in the face of adversity. It is not core purpose or meaning that matters so much as the ability for the parts of the self to continue engaging in the processes and activities they normally engage in, at a sufficient level to be able to engage well. Maintaining functioning in various areas of the self and in various life domains is seen as critical for a person to be able to be resilient.

Adversity can present significant obstacles that can easily shut down a person's ability to function in various ways, creating mental or physical impairments, psychological impairments, impairments in one's social interactions and social relationships, and difficulties with participating in various life activities like work or school. Being able to maintain functioning, at least to some degree and in at least some areas, does seem important in the process of dealing with significant change. However, adversity can impair functioning in ways that a person is sometimes unable to overcome. Then the challenge is to learn how to cope with this impaired functioning, such as through accommodation, adjustment, or adaptation.

Accepting one's limitations of functioning can be necessary yet challenging. A person may want to resist these limitations, but resistance sometimes does not lead to improved functioning, only frustration. To avoid frustration, acceptance may be necessary. Acceptance does not mean giving up. It means letting go of one's desire for outcomes that one cannot control. Acceptance often requires a person to recognize what they can control in a situation so they can exert control over the areas they can while letting go of those they can't control. Adjusting to the situation by changing oneself as the situation calls one to do, making claims on others for accommodations, and adapting by finding tools and means that enable one to do what one wishes given the constraints one is under are all important corollaries to acceptance.

While adversity can cause impaired functioning, it can also be an occasion for enhanced functioning. Sometimes the ways that a person learns to cope with their situation causes them to learn new skills and knowledge; to have access to more tools, resources, and support; and to find opportunities that they did not have before. These can all help a person to function better in various life domains than they did before, as well as to have increased agency and autonomy and increased well-being. While maintaining functioning is a good goal in dealing with adversity, sometimes a person is able to actually increase their functioning in some ways.

The process of overcoming adversity often has effects on functioning. Focusing on how a person functions in various aspects of life through adversity is thus an important aspect of improving resilience. By maintaining one's ability to function in at least some ways through life challenges, by accepting and coping with impaired functioning, or by enhancing functioning in some ways, a person can deal with challenges successfully. Part of increasing a person's resilience has to involve maximizing their ability to function, and helping them to adapt to changes in functioning despite the limitations brought about by adversity.

Being able to maintain or improve functioning or to adapt to limited functioning in various areas requires both internal and external resources. Some of the factors necessary for maximizing functioning include psychological traits and skills, the exercise of certain virtues, physical and mental health, social support, material resources, spiritual resources, and opportunities to engage in various practices and activities. The following chapters elaborate on many of these factors.

POSITIVE ADAPTATION

In the psychological literature, resilience is often understood as positive adaptation, or coping with change productively. Resilience is often discussed in the context of recovery and sustainability. John W. Reich, Alex J. Zautra, and John Stuart Hall define recovery as "the ability to rebound from stress" and sustainability as "the continuation of the recovery trajectory, and even growth and enhancement of function as a result of health reactions to the stressful experience."[26] Resilience, in turn, is understood as successful adaptation[27] or positive adaptation when exposed to risk.[28] The resilience paradigm normalizes positive reactions to stress, seeing positive reactions as more common among people (and communities) than negative reactions.[29]

In this view, coping with stress positively is understood in terms of adaptation: changing oneself as necessary in relation to changes in the environment in order to be able to deal with those environmental changes. Coping with stress thus requires not necessarily changing the stressors, by taking control over the factors leading to stress, but rather changing oneself. Perhaps this emphasis was developed in recognition that often we do not have control over the stressors in our lives to which we are forced to react, and so trying to control them would be frustrating and fruitless. What we can control, as Stoics famously recognized, is ourselves. In order to be resilient, this self-change has to be positive, meaning that it benefits a person rather than harming them, by increasing rather than decreasing their basic human capacities, including their agency, autonomy, and meaning-making capacity. This, in turn, improves their well-being and functioning.

Change is not always productive. While positive adaptation is ideal, people sometimes change in response to adversity in ways that are negative. For example, they can develop negative psychological states, unhealthy coping mechanisms, vices, and negative attitudes, and their personalities can become harsh, judgmental, obsessive, or fearful. Consider the way someone who has been bullied or abused can come to develop the traits of their bully or abuser. Dealing with adversity can also lead to diminished functioning and decreased agency and autonomy, as when a person feels beaten down by the system that wrongs them.

Positive adaptation, on the other hand, involves developing positive psychological states, healthy coping mechanisms, positive attitudes, and virtues. Personalities can flower and flourish; a person can develop knowledge and wisdom, greater empathy and respect for others, tenderness, gentleness, and understanding. While negative change harms a person in various ways, positive change increases well-being, enhances empathy and understanding, promotes meaning, increases functioning in various life activities, enhances agency and autonomy, and makes it easier for a person to interact with others and the world.

Positive adaptation requires both internal and external capacities. Internal capacities include virtues like courage and inner strength, attitudes such as optimism and hope, and skills like emotional regulation and flexibility. External capacities include resources like healthcare access and support like family and other social networks. A person cannot simply will themselves to be resilient; they have to have sufficient resources, support, and opportunities to be able to exercise resilience.

Positive adaptation is not only about adjusting to circumstances, but also about learning new skills and capacities that allow one to manage circumstances. Being able to adjust to difficult circumstances can enable a person to deal with these circumstances successfully so the adversity does not overwhelm them or rule their life. But being able to modify one's circumstances—not just oneself, but the situation one is in—is also often important. While learning how to adjust to a situation is important, learning how to make the situation more manageable is as well. This often requires learning new skills and techniques and developing new capacities and virtues that allow a person to manage their situation so they have more control over it. Positive adaptation describes the positive growth that a person undergoes as they learn how to manage or adjust to circumstances as needed. This enables them to maximize their functioning in various life domains and involves exercising—and consequently improving—their core capacities for agency, autonomy, and meaning-making.

In a virtuous circle, positive adaptation and basic human capacities are conducive to each other. Having adequate agency, autonomy, and meaning-making capacity increases a person's ability to be resilient, but being resilient also increases agency, autonomy, and meaning-making. Both resilience and capacities of agency, autonomy, and meaning-making are thus transactional with each other, where each helps to co-constitute the other.[30]

Resilience involves having adequate agency, autonomy, and meaning-making capacities and being able to mobilize these to address difficulties through managing or adjusting to them, in a way that consequently also increases these core capacities. Developing greater resilience thus requires interventions that promote autonomy, agency, and meaning-making, at the same time that it improves these. Through exercising agency, autonomy, and meaning-making, a person can maintain their integrity as a human being, fulfilling the core functions of a human being, as well as function in various areas that are important to a human life.

An Account of Resilience, So Far

Resilience involves at least partly positive adaptation, or changing oneself in ways that enable a person to manage or adjust to their circumstances while maximizing their functioning. It involves exercising—and often improving—agency, autonomy, and meaning-making, some of the core aspects of being human. Resilience does not always or necessarily require achieving equilibrium or stability, though it may; sometimes resilience is about being able to adapt continuously to continuous change. Adaptation is positive when it involves maintaining or increasing functioning in various life domains and maintaining or increasing core functioning as a human being—in other words, enhancing agency, autonomy, and meaning-making as much as possible. Adaptation that decreases functioning by shutting a person down, such as in the case of adopting unhealthy coping methods or developing a harsher, more pessimistic personality, is not positive and does not constitute resilience.

Resilience requires changing oneself to deal with or manage circumstances in a way that maximizes basic human capacities like agency, autonomy, and meaning-making—and consequently functioning and well-being—given the constraints of the situation. By enabling a person to exercise these key components of being human, resilience allows a person to maintain integrity as a human being. A person may undergo significant change and transformation in the process of positive adaptation, but what they will not change is their identity as a human being. In other words, an individual's personal identity may change considerably in response to difficulties, but their identity as a human being is constant. However, the more resilient they are, the more able they will be to participate in practices that are constitutive of what it is to be human. The capacities to exercise agency, autonomy, and meaning-making are especially critical components of resilience, enabling a person to deal with adverse situations. At the same time, resilient behaviors increase these core capacities, enabling a person to thrive as a human being even in the face of obstacles.[31]

Resilience is not a single skill, capacity, or attitude but rather a set of skills, capacities, and attitudes. Mianna Lotz describes resilience as "a global and general capacity—not a single trait or attribute but, rather, *a suite or cluster of skills, attitudes, and resources which constitute a general disposition and orientation* towards the world and one's place and condition within it."[32] This general disposition and orientation is one of learning and growth, of being able to be better in some way—as a human being, and as a particular individual—than one was before. Lotz suggests that resilience encompasses something broader than just a response to adversity. She says that resilience is not only relevant to those who have experienced significant adversity "but also is essential for every human agent in the pursuit of a flourishing life," given that we strive to pursue goals and desires that go beyond our present capacity.[33] Resilience is how we respond to life events in general, not just the kind of bad events that constitute adversity and challenge.

Resilience should not be understood as primarily backward-looking, aiming to return to a baseline state, but rather forward-looking, aiming to adapt continuously, as needed, to perpetual changes. This is captured in the related concept of sustainability, introduced earlier. Rather than looking backward at a previous baseline to which a system or person tries to return, sustainability focuses on looking forward at a future goal that enables the system or person to endure through future changes. In the context of systems, Kelly Parker and Daniel Brunson define sustainability as "the capacity of a social system (including its physical and economic foundations) to continue to meet people's needs into the indefinite future."[34]

In a psychological context, resilience as sustainability is about pushing forward, learning, and growing. The goal of resilience should not be simply absence of harm or risk (melioration of adversity), as Alex J. Zautra, John Stuart Hall, and Kate E. Murray argue, "but also capacity, thoughtfulness, planning, and a forward-leaning orientation that includes attainable goals and a realistic vision for the community as a whole."[35] Mere survival is insufficient for resilience; achieving well-being and flourishing is also necessary. Resilience is not just about neutralizing the effects of adversity, but rather about learning and growing in response to adversity. Resilience as sustainability is about flourishing as a human being, in part by developing core capacities for agency, autonomy, and meaning-making.

Sometimes resilience requires changing oneself in response to a situation, especially when one is powerless over the situation, and sometimes it requires changing the situation, when one has the ability, so that it becomes more manageable. Knowing when one's actions can make a difference and employing one's energies effectively are important in being able to discern when it is appropriate to try to change a situation versus when it is appropriate to try to accept a situation over which one has no control. Accepting a situation requires adjusting one's attitudes, expectations, and actions in relation to the difficult situation. Resilience sometimes involves accepting what one has no control over and doing what one can to make the best of a bad situation, while sometimes it involves figuring out how to change a situation over which one has some, though perhaps very little, control.

As a way of coping with adversity, resilience is one way—along with skills and capacities such as setting and working toward goals, seeking out help, and engaging in social interaction—of responding to the myriad vulnerabilities that people with mental illness face, which I describe in chapter 2. Some of the components of resilience include having a positive attitude, in particular an attitude of optimism and hope, an ability to face one's fear without trying to escape from it, having cognitive and emotional flexibility, possessing creativity in finding alternative ways to do what one wants to do given the constraints of a situation, power in changing a situation, facility in adjusting one's expectations, and finding a sense of meaning and purpose in what one does and in what happens to oneself. Some qualities that contribute to resilience include having an ethical code, a sense of spirituality, social support, role models, and both physical health and mental health.[36] Resilience requires both inner resources such as strengths, capacities, skills, and virtues, which can be developed from within through practice and participation in moral and epistemic activities; and external resources, support, and opportunities that are provided by social institutions that have as at least part of their role to empower people and protect them from vulnerability. Some of these components of resilience are developed in a mental health context in the following chapters.

Objections to the Resilience Framework

As a way of coping with adversity, resilience is one way of responding to the multitude of vulnerabilities that people with mental illness face. A resilience framework locates responsibility for dealing with adversity to the individuals experiencing adversity. It provides a way to understand what it is to "cope" with difficulties in a way that helps a person to function in various areas and to flourish as a human being. The models used to understand resilience often frame response to adversity as an individualistic behavior performed by the person experiencing adversity.

While in the psychological literature resilience is seen as a positive attribute, a characteristic or set of skills that humans should develop in order to live better lives, some critics object to the conception of resilience as too individualistic and too focused on personal growth. One criticism has to do with the way dealing with adversity is sometimes framed as a necessary process of growth. The idea that a person needs to undergo difficulties to develop positive attributes and become a better person is troubling, because it implies that going through difficulties is not only necessary, but good. It might even suggest to some that a person should seek out adversity in order to have an experience from which they can grow.

However, as Kelly Parker and Daniel Brunson point out, resilience should not imply an obligation to seek out adversity.[37] Resilience is a way that a person deals with difficulties that they can't help experiencing; difficulties should not be sought out *in order* to deal with them. There are other ways to grow besides dealing with adversity. When a person encounters adversity, they should try to cope through resilience in order to not let adversity overwhelm them, but when a person wants to grow and develop as a person, they should seek out other, more positive kinds of experiences from which they can grow.

Lotz's suggestion that resilience is not only about how we face harms but also a broader process of how we try to achieve our goals is helpful here. Resilience should be understood as how we face everything that we do: by exercising our capacities for autonomy, agency, and meaning-making in ways that further increase these capacities; by changing either our situation or ourselves, depending on what is required and what we have the power to do. Everything that we do is a potential site for growth, not only places where we experience adversity.

A deeper objection to resilience is that it is conceptualized in a way that is too individualistic. The framework of resilience locates the problem in the individual's experience and focuses on what the individual can and ought to do in reaction to their personal experience. It suggests that a person needs to draw on inner resources that come chiefly from themselves, such as strengths, capacities, skills, and virtues. This framework ignores the social context of adversity, social responsibility for addressing adversity, what social responses look like, the importance of having external resources to draw upon, and the social context for developing inner resources.

The resilience framework is individualistic in that it locates adversity as a problem of the individual's own experience. Katie Aubrecht observes that in the traditional resilience model of positive adaptation to adverse circumstances, "helplessness and powerlessness, in this formulation, are not matters of social justice, but of individual responsibility and capacities."[38] This can be understood in several ways.

First, the resilience framework can be individualistic in that it sometimes locates the cause of adversity in the individual. Martin Huth notes that the causes of adversity are often seen in binary terms, where adversity is sometimes naturalized and seen as mere misfortune, due to the way nature (and, in the case of mental illness, the body and brain) is structured, or sometimes seen as a natural consequence of bad actions the person themselves or someone else undertook.[39] In the latter, the person themselves or some other specifiable agent is seen as having caused the adversity.

When specific agents can be identified as causing the problem, control and responsibility are understood in a liability model. In this view, if the problem was in the control of some identifiable agent, then that agent is blameworthy, and it is that agent's responsibility to address it. When it is the person themselves who acted badly, they are seen as causing their own misfortune, and they are seen as blameworthy for it. In any of these scenarios, control and responsibility are assigned to the individual suffering from adversity, to other agents that acted badly, or to no one at all.

When causes of adversity are more complicated, however, the resilience model and traditional (liability) models of responsibility tend to be unhelpful. The resilience model often does not have a way to understand causes of adversity that are social or structural, for example mental illness that is due to social burdens that cause chronic stress like poverty, discrimination, or marginalization. The resilience model tends to have an impoverished view of causation of adversity.

A second way that the resilience framework is individualistic is that it suggests that the responsibility for dealing with adversity falls entirely upon the individual, who is required to change themselves in order to deal with their personal experience. Change is assumed to be within the scope of a person's agency, something they can accomplish if they only try hard enough. The resilience framework supports the belief that individuals can be resilient if they have the skills, encouragement, willpower, and motivation to do so. This unfairly burdens the person experiencing adversity.

David Harper and Ewen Speed note, "The onus for recovery is on the individual, whereby that individual must change their attitudes, values, feelings, goals, skills and roles, in a deeply personal way, in order to effect change within their own life. Rather than effecting social change, the marginalized other is required to change their personal outlook."[40] The resilient person is expected to change their beliefs, emotions, and thoughts in order to be more hopeful and health-oriented, to reflect their values (exercising autonomy), and to enable them to act as they choose (exercising agency). Harper and Speed note that this individualistic understanding of coping with adversity makes distress a problem of the diseased individual rather than a social problem involving structural inequalities.[41]

In addition to unfairly burdening the individual experiencing adversity, the concept of resilience falsely identifies the responsibility for addressing resilience as belonging to the individual facing adversity rather than to social institutions like organizations, government agencies, and systems. This ignores both the role that some social institutions may have played in creating adversity, as well as the role that social institutions can play in aiding individuals even when they played no causal role due to their greater power and capacity. Focusing on the responsibility of the individual, the resilience model leads to an impoverished view of responsibility.[42]

The concept of resilience fits a neoliberal understanding of the individual as the locus of control and responsibility, where what happens to an individual is ultimately up to them. In this neoliberal framework, individuals are "responsibilized" consumers who have the responsibility to consume the goods and services (such as healthcare) necessary to achieve the self-control and personal transformation involved with mastering one's circumstances.[43] Through this mastery, they can control what happens to them and thus have ultimate control over adversities that would otherwise threaten them with harm.

Critics trace the resilience framework for dealing with difficulties to the positive psychology movement, in which the development of personal strengths and capacities is recommended to be able to deal with life's problems.[44] The positive psychology movement supports a neoliberal economic agenda in which the responsibility for dealing with problems is outsourced to individuals, because getting individuals to do the work of dealing with problems is cheaper and easier than finding social solutions that society needs to provide. Alison Howell and Jijian Voronka observe:

> These changes [the development of the resilience and recovery frameworks] are deeply tied to broader austerity measures: getting citizens to be resilient in the face of challenges is not only cheap (in that it diverts patients out of public health care systems, in favour of self-help and positive thinking), it is also about aspiring to create a resilient citizenry, able to cope with uncertainty. This is a technology of looking inward: rather than confronting austerity measures or other matters of social justice through political action, citizens are enjoined to look inward, gather their strengths, and be resilient. Recovery and resilience, then, are notions deeply embedded with both the economic and the social imperatives of contemporary neoliberalism.[45]

In outsourcing the work of dealing with adversity to the individuals experiencing adversity, the resilience model serves the social and economic agenda of neoliberalism.

In the context of responsibility for addressing adversity faced by students, universities use the resilience model to frame responsibility for student well-being on the students themselves. Katie Aubrecht argues that universities use the resilience framework to avoid having to solve problems in the way the university is organized socially and the effects of uncertainty on students' lives. She says, "Vocabularies of resilience operate as insurance for the university against critique that the social organization of everyday life and distribution of resources within the university contribute to suffering and to the appearance and experience of uncertainty (represented as depression and anxiety) in students' lives."[46] She argues that the use of this framework occurs in a neoliberal context in which universities compete for student customers to access their product (gaining an education).

Using the resilience framework in this way has the effect of outsourcing the responsibility of helping students cope with change and difficulty onto the students themselves rather than on the institutional structures in which they find themselves. This outsourcing positions students as entrepreneurs, owners of their own business in which they pursue their interests as students. Aubrecht argues, "In encouraging students to self-monitor, regulate and manage, and in effect become their own entrepreneurs knowing when and where to seek help and refer others, the language of resilience offers a means of financial (de)regulation within the university."[47] The resilience framework helps universities cope with having diminished resources to help students by outsourcing responsibility onto the students.

Other institutions that adopt the resilience model as a way of framing responsibility for addressing adversity outsource responsibility similarly on the people facing adversity rather than framing responsibility as the work of social institutions. This allows institutions to evade responsibilities that they have, even when they helped cause the situations of adversity that people face. By outsourcing responsibility to address adversity on the individuals facing the adversity, institutions ignore both the social and structural causes of adversity, where institutions play causal roles, and the role of institutions within a responsive state, where institutions have positive obligations to aid and protect people based on their power and capacity.

Even when social institutions do not play a role in *creating* adversity, they may still play an important role in aiding individuals to *deal with* adversity. One of the roles of social institutions is to help protect individuals from various vulnerabilities they face, helping individuals to secure access to the goods to which they have a human right, providing assistance to individuals in need, and enabling civil liberties that empower individuals. Moving responsibility to address adversity from social institutions to the individuals facing adversity is a way of stripping social institutions of their power and reappropriating their role so that they no longer protect individuals from vulnerability. Outsourcing responsibility to deal with difficulties onto the individuals facing these difficulties changes the role of social institutions that were originally designated to protect individuals from vulnerability.

In addition, by locating control and responsibility within the individual, the resilience framework ignores the social context that enables people to cope with their circumstances, whether through opportunities and external resources or through inner resources. In its tendency to focus on inner resources such as strengths, capacities, skills, and virtues, the resilience framework ignores the importance of external resources, not only psychosocial resources like therapy and family, but also social resources and opportunities like jobs, education, and healthcare access. Often, people can only be resilient when they have external resources and opportunities to draw upon.

Moreover, to the extent that people are able to draw on inner resources like strengths, capacities, and skills, they are only able to do so because they have developed these strengths, capacities, and skills within a social context. Only by participating in moral and epistemic practices with others in a moral or epistemic community do we develop moral and epistemic strengths, capacities, and skills; only by practicing capacities and skills through our interactions with others do we develop these. Inner resources are always developed within a social, relational context of interacting with others and forming social relationships with others. Ignoring this social context leads to an impoverished understanding of the inner resources involved with resilience.

In addition, the emphasis on resilience obscures the important social and political role that resistance can play. Sometimes what is needed in a situation of adversity is not to change the person facing adversity so they can better deal with their situation, but rather to change the situation itself or to challenge the institutions that are responsible for creating the situation. Rather than resilience, then, sometimes the best response to adversity is resistance.[48] Resistance is a political response to a problem that is social, political, or economic. In replacing the role of resistance with resilience, the resilience framework obscures the social, political, and economic nature of many of the problems vulnerable individuals have to deal with. This masks the social, political, and economic responsibility that institutions, systems, and structures have in perpetuating and addressing the problem. Refocusing attention to the institutions and structures that helped create and maintain conditions of adversity requires us to resist and challenge these systems rather than to promote change within the self.

How Resilience Should Be Understood

In light of these objections, the concept of resilience needs to be reconceptualized to take into account the social contexts of how adversity is caused; who has responsibility to address it; how people develop the characteristics they need to deal with adversity; and what resources, support, and opportunity people need to mobilize in their efforts. I propose reconceptualizing resilience as not simply positive adaptation to difficult circumstances, through which one maintains or increases core functioning of agency, autonomy, and meaning-making, but also incorporating the idea of having adequate resources, support, and opportunity to make positive adaptation possible. Resilience involves the capacity to mobilize adequate resources, support, and opportunities effectively to cope with adversity and challenges—or, more broadly, to pursue whatever goals one has—in a manner that enables one to flourish as a human being, increasing core capacities of agency, autonomy, and meaning-making, thereby enabling functioning and well-being.

Dealing with adversity can involve changing the situation or changing oneself, whatever seems appropriate given the circumstances, depending on how much control a person is able to exert over the situation. Changing the situation can comprise an act of resistance in which one challenges the power of the institutions and systems responsible for the situation. It reconfigures the power relationship involved with the situation so that the individual can gain control over the situation rather than being overwhelmed by it. Changing oneself can involve adjusting one's expectations, accepting what one has no control over, and developing adaptations by devising alternative ways to do what one wishes given the constraints of the situation. Coping with difficulties can constitute any or all of these responses. What is best in a given situation depends on what the situation seems to call for and how much control and power a person has in relation to the situation. Sometimes this requires multiple concurrent responses rather than any single response.

The ability to mobilize resources and support and to take advantage of available opportunities is a capacity that one can have to a greater or lesser amount, depending on how much power a person has; what skills they possess that enable them to wield this power; and what resources, opportunities, and support are available. This capacity is an ability that anyone could acquire if they had the right resources, support, and opportunities to do so, and if they had sufficient experience of participating in epistemic and moral practices that allow them to develop the requisite power and skills. This participation necessarily has a social context; it must occur with other participants in an epistemic or moral community of those who recognize the legitimacy of one's participation and the moral standing and credibility of the participant.

Having the right resources, support, and opportunities is thus critical. A person can only mobilize and take advantage of what is available to them; if they do not have sufficient resources, support, and opportunities, then all the power and skills in the world will be insufficient to make a difference. Resources, support, and opportunities are social goods that are available in the social world; they are not individual goods that one could construct oneself. Thus, the social world has to be up to the task of creating and making these goods available. Social institutions must be designed so that they have and can carry out as at least one of their roles to provide resources, support, and opportunities for individuals who are in need. Individuals need a supportive society, with supportive institutions, to give them the resources, opportunities, and tools to be resilient.

Mobilizing resources and support involves recognizing and identifying relevant resources and sources of support, and using these resources and support in ways that generate success in coping with difficulties, whatever "coping with" consists of. In other words, if a situation calls for a person to accept what they cannot control, they have to be able to draw on external resources and support (along with inner resources, of course) to be successful at accepting what they cannot change. Taking advantage of opportunities involves identifying what opportunities are available to a person, and using these opportunities to deal with difficulties as the situation requires. But sufficient resources, support, and opportunities have to be available for a person to be able to mobilize and take advantage of them.

Many different kinds of resources and support can be relevant. Inner resources include strengths, capacities, skills, and virtues, as well as the possession of willpower and motivation. Spiritual resources include sources of spirituality that inspire optimism, hope, compassion, and possibility. Epistemic resources include the ability to understand one's situation and one's place and role within it, accurately and realistically. Material resources include money and materials needed to develop adaptations or to change a situation, and access to healthcare needed to maximize physical and mental health. Support includes efforts involved with caring about, helping, and protecting people, as well as providing encouragement and opportunities (especially opportunities for social interaction and social relationships) to develop capacities that help a person be better at something than they previously were. All kinds of resources and support can be relevant to being able to deal with difficulties effectively.

Opportunities include jobs, education, and various activities that give individuals ways to participate in life domains and have power and control in areas of their life. Opportunities to participate in various activities enable the development of skills, capacities, strengths, and virtues, as people develop these things by practicing them over time in a community of others who recognize one's practice as legitimate. Opportunities thus enable resources to be developed and skills, capacities, and virtues to be available to a person by being developed and exercisable.

Some of the support, resources, and opportunities that are needed can be provided interpersonally through one's relationships with other individuals, as I explain in chapter 3. However, social institutions and communities are necessary to provide many of the needed resources, support, and opportunities, as I discuss in chapters 4 and 5. Material resources usually need to come from the community, or more specifically from social institutions that have greater resources, as individuals often have inadequate material resources compared to their need. In the context of mental health, material resources include access to the mental healthcare that people with mental illness need. Institutions like churches and art communities, and public resources like open-space (natural) areas enable the development of spiritual resources and resources needed for meaning-making. Epistemic resources require a community in which a person can test the reality of their perception and understanding of the world and of themselves in relation to that of others. Efforts of caring, protecting, helping, and encouraging, as well as providing opportunities to develop capacities, skills, strengths, and virtues, require a community in which individuals and institutions alike can provide care, protection, help, and opportunities for social interaction and engagement. The community and, more particularly, social institutions that are specifically designed for this must provide opportunities like jobs, education, and places where various life activities can occur, as a person cannot usually provide these to themselves on their own.

To the extent that resilience requires external resources, support, and opportunities, people can be resilient to a greater or lesser degree depending on their privilege. Privilege enables access to these, enabling those who are situated in positions of greater privilege to have greater external resources, support, and opportunities to draw upon and take advantage of. Increasing access to these social goods requires challenging systems of privilege to make privilege more available to all and access more widespread.

Resilience also requires social uptake and responsivity, as I discuss in chapter 6. When individuals deal with their adversity by expressing their needs, voicing their concerns, or resisting unjust structures, institutions must listen. They must afford vulnerable individuals epistemic competence and credibility and be willing to be responsive to individuals' needs, concerns, and justice demands. To be responsive, institutions must be open to the possibility of change and be willing to change as needed in order to meet individuals' needs and create justice. Individuals only have power to change their situation when they have opportunities to express themselves and be heard in a way that is appropriately responsive. To be empowered to make changes that underpin socially supportive resilience practices, individuals must have the political means to work collectively in interacting with relevant institutions. Individual power is predicated on institutional power that enables individuals to have a voice and to act.

Conclusion

Saks and Steele showed resilience in many places in their lives when they faced tremendous obstacles with their mental illnesses yet managed to find ways to continue living despite illness. When faced with significant challenges, they found ways to transform their situation, when they had some control over it, or themselves, when they had to adjust and adapt to situations outside their control. As we see in future chapters, they needed considerable social support, resources, and opportunities to be successful in this. While they had inner resources they could draw on, these were insufficient by themselves to enable Saks and Steele to face their challenges with resilience. Support, resources, and opportunities from other individuals and institutions were also necessary to develop and channel their inner resources as well as to provide the means for effective response to their adversity.

Resilience is a characteristic or process that enables individuals to address their own situations of adversity by changing the situation, themselves, or both. The resilience framework provides one way to understand what kind of response is needed to address adversity, but in its traditional form it provides an impoverished view of causation of adversity and responsibility for addressing it, as well as an impoverished view of what individuals need to be able to confront their challenges and how they develop the requisite skills, virtues, and capacities. Instead of understanding resilience simply as the capacity for the individual to adapt positively to change, we should understand resilience as the capacity to mobilize resources, support, and opportunities to transform their situation or themselves (or both) in a way that increases their core functions of agency, autonomy, and meaning-making.

In the next chapter, I delineate what vulnerabilities people with mental illness have due to their illness and their position in society, showing that many of the vulnerabilities to which they are subject are social vulnerabilities that can only be addressed in a social context. Understanding the vulnerabilities individuals face helps us to understand what kinds of interventions are necessary and effective to help individuals cope, and in particular what kinds of support, resources, and opportunities individuals need to be resilient. Following this, in the rest of this book, I explore some of the support, resources, and opportunities that individuals need that must be provided by society, and in many cases by institutions (organizations and agencies) and systems that are designed to provide these. Let us now examine the vulnerabilities that people with mental illness are subject to so we can better understand what they need to be able to cope with their challenges in a resilient way.

Chapter 2

Vulnerabilities of Mental Illness

Introduction

People who have mental illness are vulnerable to many harms because of their illness and face special challenges in trying to overcome their illness. For example, consider Elyn Saks's life story. A law professor at the University of Southern California, Saks also has schizophrenia. In her memoir, *The Center Cannot Hold*, Saks describes being an intellectually gifted young woman, with an intense work ethic, who was overcome by voices in her head giving her commands to act in ways that made her appear "crazy." The voices came on slowly, but as they grew more anchored in her mind, Saks spent years of her young adulthood in and out of hospitals while being treated for psychosis.

A promising young scholar, she won a prestigious Marshall Scholarship to study classics at Oxford University as a graduate student. There, the unease she had felt as a teenager morphed into full-blown psychosis. Academic study provided a way for her to focus her mind while fighting delusions, and she managed to get accepted into Yale Law School. However, while being tormented by delusions, hallucinations, and severe cognitive disorganization, her psychosis worsened to the point where she had to drop out of law school after only a few short months because she was hospitalized for such a long time. Eventually, she was diagnosed with paranoid schizophrenia.

After a year of hospitalizations and medication changes, she was able to put her life back together and return to law school, and she managed to finish out her time in school without having to be hospitalized again.

She continued to struggle with psychosis, however, and felt like she was battling it constantly. After graduating law school, she got a job as a lawyer with the Connecticut Legal Services before embarking on her academic career, which allowed her more flexibility to deal with her mental health challenges than her job as a traditional lawyer.

When Saks was diagnosed with paranoid schizophrenia, she struggled with coming to terms with what the diagnosis meant. Like many people in the Western world, she held stereotypes about severe mental illness that made her want to reject her diagnosis. She describes her fears of what her life would be as a result of schizophrenia:

> And then there was the whole mythology of schizophrenia, aided and abetted by years of books and movies that presented people like me as hopelessly evil or helplessly doomed. I would become violent, as the delusions in my head grew more real to me than reality itself. My psychotic episodes would increase, and last longer; my intelligence would be severely compromised. Maybe I'd end my life in an institution; maybe I'd *live* my life in an institution. Or become homeless, a bag lady whose family could no longer care for her. I'd be that wild-eyed character on the city sidewalk that all the nice baby carriage-pushing mommies shrink away from. *Get away from the crazy lady.* I'd love no one; no one would love me.[1]

She further summarizes many of the losses she thought she would experience: "The prognosis: I would largely lose the capacity to care for myself. I wasn't expected to have a career, or even a job that might bring in a paycheck. I wouldn't be able to form attachments, or keep friendships, or find someone to love me, or have a family of my own—in short, I'd never have a *life*."[2] As schizophrenia is a severe mental illness, often with a negative prognosis, manageable but not curable, and causing tremendous harms and losses, Saks was understandably afraid of what her future life could look like.

Saks's fears of what her future life would be like were not unfounded. Stereotypes of what schizophrenia looks like rest on actual data of what life is like for many people who have schizophrenia. We are all familiar with homeless people who mutter to themselves or shout incoherently to nobody. Many people with schizophrenia are homeless or incarcerated; nearly a third of the population of chronically homeless people have severe mental illness,[3] and about half of all inmates do.[4] The highest concentration of inmates with severe mental illness are housed in jails, where they frequently serve time for petty crimes related to their illness or to being homeless, such as being a nuisance or urinating in public. While hospital beds for psychiatric patients are scarce, people with severe mental illness are nonetheless sometimes hospitalized for months at a time, and some people cycle in and out of hospitals continuously (sometimes alternating with bouts of homelessness). Saks's fears that she could wind up homeless, in jail, or institutionalized for the long term were not unreasonable, based on what life is actually like for many people with schizophrenia.

Ken Steele was a man who had schizophrenia who lived the kind of life Saks feared. (He died in 2000.) His memoir, *The Day the Voices Stopped*, details his difficult life story.[5] He was diagnosed with paranoid schizophrenia when he was a teenager and spent over three decades rotating through hospitalizations, long-term institutionalizations in state psychiatric facilities (lasting months at a time), and homelessness. Constantly he heard voices, except when he was too sedated on very high doses of first-generation antipsychotic medications (medications like Thorazine and Haldol). His voices were usually disparaging, encouraging him daily to kill himself.

Psychiatrist Stephen Mark Goldfinger, who later worked with Steele after he had recovered from his mental illness, recalls meeting Steele for the first time when he was living on the streets in San Francisco: "I have no real memory of that first encounter—Ken was just one of the hundreds of foul-smelling, unshaven, psychologically disorganized men and women I worked with day after day. Most were on the streets, in desperate exile forced on them by overpowering voices and hallucinations. As a psychiatrist, I did what I could to help, but I faced the depressing reality that many of them would live out their lives in institutions or, worse, return to the streets."[6] Steele fit the stereotype of the unkempt, homeless person with severe mental illness who talks overtly with his voices.

For decades, Steele had a very hard time coping with his voices and suffered many harms from his schizophrenia, including not only long-term institutionalization and homelessness, but also exploitation, violence, abuse, trauma, and coercion. When young, he was easy to take advantage of. While trying to make a life for himself in New York City as a young adult, he was groomed for sexual exploitation and abuse, which exacerbated his voices, made him actively suicidal, and led to his first hospitalization.

While hospitalized and institutionalized during these three decades, he was put in seclusion for weeks at a time, tied up in restraints for much of the time he was in seclusion, and given injections of medication against his will. In some institutions, he was subject to violence and abuse by other psychiatric patients. Steele depicts this violence in his description of one of his hospitalization stays: "The ward to which I was eventually assigned was full of the most dangerous patients, and they attacked in groups. Behind the safety of their glass-paned nursing station, staff members could be seen smiling and laughing as patients pummeled one another. It seemed to me that some aides even wagered on winners and losers."[7] His experience fit the traditional stereotype of what being institutionalized was like, popularized by media such as the movie *One Flew Over the Cuckoo's Nest*.

While homeless, Steele lived as many homeless people do: on the streets, camping out in parks when he could, covering himself with leaves for a blanket, relying on missions and soup kitchens for food. An avid reader (he had been a top student when he was young, similar to Saks), he found solace in the public library. After being homeless for a while, his voices would compel him to try to commit suicide, and his troubling behavior got the attention of law enforcement, who hospitalized him. In this way, he cycled through homelessness and institutionalization. Many of his experiences traumatized him. For a long time, Steele lived a tragic life that would be undesirable to anyone.

People with severe mental illness are vulnerable to many harmful conditions. As Saks recognized, they have a strong chance of winding up homeless, incarcerated, or institutionalized for long periods of time. They are prone to being shunned, stigmatized, and discriminated against. They are more likely to be unemployed or underemployed, with less than a quarter with severe mental illness employed even though almost three-quarters express an interest in working.[8] In part because they often cannot obtain adequate employment, people with severe mental illness also tend to be poor, with nearly 40 percent having annual incomes of less than $10,000.[9]

As we see from Steele's experience, other harms that people with mental illness are vulnerable to include exploitation, abuse, trauma, and coercion. Research shows that mental illness is a cue for sexual exploitation[10] as well as for other types of exploitation such as financial exploitation and cheating.[11] People with mental illness experience high rates of various types of victimization, including theft, physical violence, and harassment.[12] People with schizophrenia have high rates of having a history of trauma or loss.[13] People are sometimes subject to abuse from either staff or fellow psychiatric patients in psychiatric facilities. Coercive treatment is common, especially when people are hospitalized involuntarily.

People who have severe mental illness are also vulnerable to many interpersonal harms. Saks describes the difficulty of making friends and even of simply having social interactions while she was overcome by voices and delusions. Because there was a huge part of herself that she thought she should keep secret, she held back a lot from other people, and it hurt her ability to become close to them. It was difficult for her to create friendships, but when she did, she treasured them immensely.

Some people lose friends when their friends do not know how to be there for the person suffering. Some people, like Steele, become estranged from family members when their family members do not accept them. After he showed signs of schizophrenia as a young man, Steele's parents wanted nothing to do with him. Later in life, after his recovery, Steele counseled parents to stay connected to their children, no matter how much they struggled, because he saw firsthand the harm that estrangement brings.

Saks notes the loneliness involved with illness. She says, "One of the worst aspects of schizophrenia is the profound isolation—the constant awareness that you're different, some sort of alien, not really human."[14] Steele also shows the deep isolation he experienced: "I was alone in this life except for my voices and imagination."[15] People who become isolated due to their illness suffer many kinds of harms. One significant harm is losing the opportunity to interact with others in ways that are important for developing and exercising agency. When people are socially isolated, they lose the opportunity to participate in shared moral and epistemic practices with other members of a moral and epistemic community, and this diminishes their agency.[16]

In addition to social and interpersonal harms, people with severe mental illness are also, of course, vulnerable to many harms to their minds and bodies. People with schizophrenia, for example, are vulnerable to false beliefs and false perceptions (delusions and hallucinations), cognitive disorganization and distortions that can override whatever intellectual abilities they have, apathy and disinterest, problems with hygiene and self-care, and social withdrawal and isolation. People with severe mental illness are more likely to have physical health conditions such as obesity, metabolic syndrome, diabetes, heart problems, and asthma, partly due to certain medications and partly due to a lack of self-care. Between not taking good care of themselves and tendencies toward suicidal ideation, people with severe mental illness also have a higher mortality rate and tend to die much younger than the general population.[17] People with severe mental illness are thus prone to many different kinds of harms both caused and exacerbated by their illness.

This chapter examines the kinds of vulnerabilities to which people with severe mental illness are subject, analyzing mental illness in a vulnerability framework that illuminates both the ways in which mental illness can harm people and the types of responses that are appropriate for addressing these harms. In this chapter, I examine what vulnerability is and the ways in which mental illness both constitutes a vulnerability and incurs other vulnerabilities, compounding and exacerbating the risk of harm individuals face. Many of these vulnerabilities are social, in that how a person is situated in relation to others and to society affects what vulnerabilities they are subject to; responses to vulnerability, therefore, must be social, too. I argue that interpersonal and institutional interventions that promote agency, autonomy, and meaning-making are necessary to address people's vulnerability. Providing adequate support, resources, and opportunities to help people increase their agency, autonomy, and meaning-making is necessary to aid people with mental illness to cope with their challenges.

Vulnerability: An Overview

Vulnerability can be understood as risk of suffering harm or adversity. Sometimes vulnerability is understood more broadly as openness to being affected by something,[18] where how one is affected may be either positive or negative, but here I want to focus on the narrower definition that identifies what is problematic about vulnerability: that it subjects someone to risk of suffering harm or adversity. Vulnerability typically involves facing threats to vital interests such as one's life, body, mind, or agency. People can have dispositional vulnerability, or the potential to be vulnerable, by being at risk of experiencing harm, or they can have occurrent vulnerability, where they are actually subject to harm. "Vulnerability" (singular) often connotes the general state of being vulnerable, while "vulnerabilities" (plural) often refers to specific vulnerabilities: specific harms or threats to which a person may be subject.

Philosophers typically distinguish vulnerability among two broad categories, which may be conceptualized in different ways. Catriona Mackenzie, Wendy Rogers, and Susan Dodds delineate two sources of vulnerability: ontological vulnerability, which is inherent to the human condition and which we thus all share by being human, and contingent vulnerability, which is experienced by particular individuals in specific contexts.[19] Martha Albertson Fineman distinguishes different types of vulnerability in a contrasting way, not in terms of their sources but in terms of their scopes, describing ontological vulnerability as universal, applying to all human beings, and contingent vulnerability as particular, applying to specific individuals or social groups based on social, historical, economic, and political factors.[20] These two sets of terms do not map onto each other neatly. Ontological vulnerability is universal when it is dispositional, as everyone has the potential to experience it, but it is particular when it is occurrent, as only some people are currently vulnerable in this way depending on what happens to them in their lives. Similarly, contingent vulnerability, or vulnerability caused by context-specific social factors, has the potential to apply to everyone if they are situated in the right ways, but in practice it only applies to those who are in fact situated in these ways. In the next section, I explicate some different forms of ontological vulnerability as well as introduce contingent vulnerability.

Ontological Vulnerability

Ontological vulnerability is the vulnerability we have by virtue of being human; it is vulnerability that is inherent to the human condition, and thus it applies to all people. All people have at least dispositional ontological vulnerability, where they have the potential to be subject to certain kinds of vulnerability by virtue of being human, although only some people experience this vulnerability occurrently, depending on what is happening to them in their lives. Ontological vulnerability is thus universal in its dispositional state—everyone has the potential to be ontologically vulnerable—but it is particular in its occurrent state, as it is only experienced by some people sometimes, depending on socially contingent factors.

Different aspects of our humanity lead to different ways we experience ontological vulnerability. Some of the kinds of ontological vulnerability I am interested in here are the vulnerability we face as embodied and en-minded subjects, the vulnerability we face living under various social structures, and the vulnerability we experience as epistemic and moral agents. Usually, ontological vulnerability is described in the literature chiefly in terms of corporeal vulnerability, or the vulnerability we have by virtue of being embodied and having bodies. Reducing ontological vulnerability to corporeal vulnerability, however, is a mentally ableist move that ignores the vulnerabilities we have that are inherent to having minds. Ontological vulnerability is comprised of mental vulnerability as well. Moreover, ontological vulnerability is not just concerned with the fragility of our minds and bodies (the ways that we are embodied and en-minded), but also with the precariousness of the institutions and structures that govern our lives, and the concepts, beliefs, desires, and values we have as epistemic and moral agents. Two additional aspects of vulnerability that are inherent to the human condition are the vulnerability we face living under various social structures, and the vulnerability we have as subjects of experience and as moral and epistemic agents. Let us look at these forms of ontological vulnerability in turn.

CORPOREAL AND MENTAL VULNERABILITY

First let us consider corporeal vulnerability. By virtue of being embodied, corporeal subjects, we are vulnerable to the frailties of being alive and being creatures who will someday die. By having bodies and being embodied, we are all vulnerable to conditions like injury, impairment, illness, and death.[21] We are born; we go through different life stages, some of which involve dependency on others (like childhood and old age); our bodies can break; our minds can deteriorate; we can gain and lose different kinds of abilities; eventually, if we are lucky enough to live long enough, our bodies will decay and die. Being embodied and en-minded makes us fragile.

Martha Albertson Fineman observes that this corporeal vulnerability is universal to all humans, because all humans are embodied. It is an inevitable part of life, and it endures throughout our lifetimes.[22] She says, "Vulnerability initially should be understood as arising from our embodiment, which carries with it the ever-present possibility of harm, injury, and misfortune from mildly adverse to catastrophically devastating events, whether accidental, intentional, or otherwise."[23] Vulnerability can be understood as "a state of constant possibility of harm"[24] and change. Corporeal vulnerability can thus be understood as vulnerability to harm and adversities that make our lives difficult based on the nature of our bodies and the fact that we are embodied.

We are not *only* embodied, however; we are also en-minded (within a mind); by this, I mean that we also have minds. Our material essence can be understood as a mind-body subject that has multiple components, including different parts and aspects of the body and different parts and aspects of the mind. The mental parts of our selves must be acknowledged in any discussion of vulnerability. Our identity and agency are predicated on the fact that we have minds that think, feel, and will. The fact that our bodies can *do* anything depends on the fact that we have minds that can consider different options, make decisions, form intentions, and will to act. It is not only our bodies that are fragile, subject to life processes, sometimes dependent on others, able to be injured or impaired, able to lose abilities, and subject to decay and death; our minds are equally fragile. We have different mental abilities at different developmental stages; our minds can break when we are subject to significant stress or mental illness; we can lose mental capacities; we can lose our sense of self, identity, and agency when our mind decays. The fragility of our minds can be understood as a sort of mental vulnerability.

Corporeal vulnerability must therefore be understood in tandem with mental vulnerability, as similar life processes apply to both. Since the mind and body are intertwined, mental vulnerability and corporeal vulnerability go hand in hand; mind and body are both subject to similar kinds of changes and losses. They are worth distinguishing as different aspects of the self, however, because each component—the mind and the body—can be injured, impaired, or dying in distinct ways.[25] Mental illness, for example, injures primarily the mind (by virtue of the mental illness symptoms associated with various diagnoses) and secondarily the body (for example by causing appetite or sleep changes): it injures both, but in different ways. Mental illness is a threat to us primarily through our mental vulnerability, but also secondarily through our corporeal vulnerability.

Mental vulnerability is just as universal a form of vulnerability as corporeal vulnerability, because all humans have minds of some sort by virtue of being human. Because humans are necessarily en-minded, all humans are vulnerable to various harms to their minds. Mental vulnerability is an ontological vulnerability we have simply by being human.

Philosophers might object to my classification of mental vulnerability as a form of ontological vulnerability, arguing that corporeal vulnerability takes into account the fragilities of our minds. They may view injury, impairment, illness, and death as processes that happen to our minds as well as our bodies, or more properly that happen to our minds alongside our bodies, as bodies and minds are necessarily intertwined. For example, traumatic brain injury is injury to the body (the physical brain) that has profound effects on the mind; physical illnesses can affect how a person thinks and feels. Nonetheless, the different harms that occur to bodies and minds are distinguishable.

While it is true that our minds and bodies are so interconnected that something cannot happen to one without affecting the other, they are nonetheless distinguishable as sites where processes occur. Consciousness, cognition, perception, rationality, emotional sensitivity and regulation, and volition can all be affected in distinctive ways that—while having a bodily aspect—do not simply reduce to the body. Ignoring the way mental processes can be harmed or believing that harms to mental processes reduce to harms of the body is a mentally ableist move that those who have the privilege to not have to consider specific harms done to the mind can afford to do. People who have had their minds harmed in certain ways recognize that mental processes can be damaged in distinctive ways.

Two forms of ontological vulnerability are thus corporeal and mental vulnerability, both of which describe fragilities we have the potential to be subject to by virtue of having certain characteristics of being human, namely of being embodied and en-minded, or of having bodies and having minds. Corporeal vulnerability describes harms that we are at risk of experiencing in relation to our bodies, while mental vulnerability describes harms that we are at risk of experiencing in relation to our minds. Our bodies can break, be hurt, lose abilities, be sick, experience different developmental stages, and die. Our minds can, too, in ways that undoubtedly affect the body (just as our bodily experiences affect the mind), yet which are distinctive enough to understand in their own way. Mental illness, dementia, stress, and anxiety are harms that we all have the potential to be subject to, by virtue of being human, although only some of us experience these at a given time depending on what has happened to us in our lives. Mental vulnerability is thus dispositionally universal and occurrently contingent, yet inherent to the human condition and thus ontological.

SOCIAL-STRUCTURAL VULNERABILITY

Another type of ontological vulnerability is social-structural vulnerability, or the susceptibility to harm that we face in having our lives governed by various social structures. As social creatures, we are embedded within social structures such as institutions, systems, communities, society, and governments that regulate and organize our lives. In this context, Judith Butler argues that the world always acts on us even as we are acting as agents.[26] In terms of epistemic agency, our concepts, language, and categories are already given to us, and we must navigate the world with the concepts, language, and categories already available to us. In terms of moral agency, we are thrown into a social world over which we have little control, subject to various social structures that provide the backdrop for, and thus condition, our experience and action.

Butler describes our inherent relationality and the way we are necessarily interdependent with each other. She says, "As I have tried to suggest by calling attention to the dual dimensions of performativity, we are invariably acted on and acting, and this is one reason performativity cannot be reduced to the idea of free, individual performance. We are called names and find ourselves living in a world of categories and descriptions way before we start to sort them critically and endeavor to change or make them our own."[27] Concepts and understandings shape our knowledge of the world and of ourselves before we even have a chance to critically engage with them.

Encountering frameworks of meaning impacts how we think about ourselves and our experiences. Dominant narratives that frame how we should understand particular kinds of experiences shape our personal understandings of our own experiences.[28] For example, dominant narratives of mental illness as a brain disease color the understanding a person with mental illness has of their own experience, as they learn to think of aspects of their experience in terms of *Diagnostic and Statistical Manual* (DSM) symptoms that have neurochemical causes and that can only or best be addressed with medication.[29] This limits a person's understanding of their mental illness experience, precluding interpersonal aspects of understanding such as how a person relates to and interacts with specific others in their lives, and shapes their self-concept as a sick person needing treatment. Or consider the way dominant narratives that stigmatize mental illness become adopted by individuals with mental illness who then internalize that stigma as self-stigma.[30] Dominant narratives, such as narratives of mental illness, are often accepted and incorporated into a person's self-understanding and self-concept before the person even has a chance to critically interrogate them.

The world is as it is before we get to act in and on it. The world is presented to us in a certain way, and we need to adapt ourselves to that world in order to make sense of it, act within it, and flourish as a human being. As social subjects, we are vulnerable to social structures that govern how we experience the world and what we can do in the world, in particular, vulnerable to the various challenges and adversities social structures present, such as inequality, oppression, domination, coercion, marginalization, exploitation, and other forms of harm and injustice. We embody a precarious position because we lack control over the way the world is structured and what the world can do to us, yet we are dependent on the world for our very existence.

More specifically, Butler argues, we are dependent on infrastructure, "understood complexly as environment, social relations, and networks of support and sustenance,"[31] or what I like to think of as structures and systems. Butler argues that it is the body that is particularly vulnerable to infrastructure, but I think it is more accurate to say that our entire selves are. She adds, "We are vulnerable to decimated or disappearing infrastructures, economic supports, and predictable and well-compensated labor."[32] We are dependent on the quality of existing social structures and systems and on whatever social, economic, and political resources exist; we are vulnerable to needing resources that may be lacking, and we are vulnerable to what is problematic, harmful, or unjust, in our social structures and systems.

This impacts our agency, both epistemic and moral. We are only able to know in relation to the concepts and language that is available to us, given by our social structures and culture. We are only able to act in relation to the institutions that structure our possibilities and motivations for action. Existing social structures and systems condition our choices and actions and thus circumscribe our agency.

Bryan Turner notes that infrastructure is intended and often serves to *protect* us from vulnerability. He says, "In order to protect themselves from the uncertainties of the everyday world, they [people] must build social institutions (especially political, familial, and cultural institutions) that come to constitute what we call 'society.'"[33] Yet while institutions are designed to protect us, they become sources of vulnerability as well. He notes, "We create institutions to reduce our vulnerability and attain security, but these institutional patterns are always imperfect, inadequate, and precarious."[34] Since social structures and system are themselves precarious, they become a source of vulnerability even as we are dependent on them to try to protect us from other vulnerabilities.

Our identity as relational beings makes us vulnerable both to each other, in an interpersonal way, and to the structures that condition our experience and action. Our need to act in the world as moral agents makes us dependent on other individuals—as we act in relation to the ways *they* act in the world—and on the social, economic, political, and environmental structures that serve as the backdrop for our actions. Our precarity is based on this relationality and dependence.

In the context of mental illness, this means that people with mental illness are dependent on the various social structures that shape their experience. These include the mental health system and general healthcare system as well as many other systems and structures, such as systems of housing and employment. As I explain in chapter 5, the quality of these structures and systems affects the opportunities and options that a person has available to them, the resources they can draw upon, the kinds of actions they can perform, and the kind of life they are capable of living. People with mental illness are dependent on—and thus vulnerable to—many structures and systems, as we all are, to provide them with possibilities for action and to enable them to live certain kinds of lives.

Vulnerability as Epistemic and Moral Subjects and Agents

Besides being embodied, en-minded, and embedded within social structures, a fourth way that we experience ontological vulnerability is by virtue of being epistemic and moral subjects and agents. We are not only dependent on the world, and on the structures and systems that exist in the world, but we are also subject to what happens in the world, and this puts us at risk of losing our ability to understand and navigate the world and our epistemic and moral agency. Simply by living in the world, we are vulnerable to experiencing epistemic and moral losses because the world can act on us in ways that we have no or limited control over. In being epistemic and moral agents, we risk losing foundational aspects of our agency; in being subjects that experience the world in epistemic and moral contexts, we risk losing our conceptual understanding and our understanding of human interaction.

Jonathan Lear describes this vulnerability as follows:

> As finite erotic creatures it is an essential part of our nature that we take risks just by being in the world. As finite creatures we are vulnerable: we may suffer physical and emotional injury, we may make significant mistakes, even the concepts with which we understand ourselves and the world may collapse—and yet as erotic creatures [reaching out to the world in desire for that which we take to be valuable, beautiful, and good] we reach out to the world and try to embrace it. For all the risks involved, we make an effort to live with others; on occasion we aspire to intimacy; we try to understand the world; on occasion we try to express ourselves and create something; we aim toward living (what we take to be) a happy life. As finite,

> erotic creatures it is a necessary aspect of our existence that our lives are marked by risk. We are familiar with the idea that we are creatures who necessarily inhabit a world. But *a world is not merely the environment in which we move about; it is that over which we lack omnipotent control, that about which we may be mistaken in significant ways, that which may intrude upon us, that which may outstrip the concepts with which we seek to understand it.* Thus living within a world has inherent and unavoidable risk.[35]

It is the fact that we inhabit a world that we do not have full control over that puts us in a position of risk with respect to what that world can do to us. The world can act upon us in ways that compromise our understanding, our subjectivity (the way we experience the world), and our agency (the way we act in the world). Simply by living in the world, we are subject to a wide array of risks that can threaten our way of being in the world. There is no way to escape these risks, as human beings must live in the world.

Living in the world thus puts us at risk by virtue of being subjects (people who experience the world) and agents (people who act in the world). Events in the world can change or eliminate our concepts, beliefs, desires, and values in ways that we have no control over, often do not understand, and sometimes do not even recognize. This has both epistemic and moral ramifications.

In an epistemic context, we can lose knowledge, be prone to misunderstanding and nonunderstanding, and experience a loss of meaning and coherence; all of these affect how a person experiences the world as a subject. In his book *Radical Hope*, Jonathan Lear shows that the Crow tribe experienced a particular form of ontological vulnerability when they experienced a loss of meaning in their conceptual awareness.[36] In their traditional way of living, as a warrior tribe, events held meaning in relation to going to battle, and people strived to live up to ideals, such as the ideal of courage, associated with being a warrior tribe and a nomadic hunting tribe. After the US government took land from the Crow and forced them to change their warrior culture into a farming culture, they lost the meaning that certain acts associated with being in battle once held, so that traditional ideals of courage no longer made sense. Since they could no longer live up to the ideals associated with traditional roles, they consequently lost their sense of identity. Events in the world changed how the Crow experienced the world, and themselves, and thus changed their identity as subjects of experience.

Lear argues that, in dealing with this loss of meaning and shift in ideals, the Crow exhibited radical hope, believing that some good will come to them even if they did not have the conceptual awareness to understand what that good would consist of. This hope allowed them to move forward from their loss and change their ideals of courage and valor, so that they could reconceptualize what it meant to be a good Crow. This required them to shift some of the desires and values they held so they no longer related to war or hunting but rather to their new life revolving around agriculture. In some ways, this changed their identity—or, at least, what it meant to be a good Crow.

What Lear's analysis shows us here is that when the world changes too dramatically, a person can lose what understanding they had of the world, and consequently themselves. Epistemic losses such as these can be very difficult to overcome and often require tremendous resources to cope with. By living in the world as subjects who experience the world, we run the risk of having our conceptual understanding change in significant ways that can affect our identity and agency.

We can thus experience significant epistemic losses as epistemic agents and subjects. Epistemic losses can include situations of hermeneutical harms, where individuals lack the hermeneutical resources to make sense of their situation, such as when they experience some kind of disordered bodily or mental experience that they do not have a name or concept for; and testimonial exclusion, when individuals' knowledge is not taken seriously so they are disbarred from participating in further epistemic activity. Hermeneutical harms and testimonial exclusion constitute injustices when they are based on identity prejudice credibility deficits.[37] For example, when mental health clinicians believe that a person is too incompetent to possess or articulate credible knowledge of their experience, simply by virtue of having mental illness, their testimony is discredited, creating testimonial injustice. When mental health clinicians fail to help a person understand their experience because they believe the person is incapable of such understanding based on having a mental illness, they commit hermeneutical injustice to the individual.

Epistemic losses can also accrue due to other types of injustices, such as the injustices involved with domination and oppression. The changes in livelihood and consequently changes in concepts and values that the Crow experienced at the hands of the U.S. government were due to systematic oppression. Marginalization, exploitation, violence, and other forms of oppression can all create epistemic losses for the people subject to them.

Epistemic losses can also occur when there is no injustice due to what happens to a person or their environment. For example, a person may lack hermeneutical resources to understand their situation simply because they lack the capacity due to an intellectual disability. Sometimes epistemic losses result after a person has initially had concepts to understand, such as a person with cognitive decline who once knew how to interact with others appropriately but no longer has the memory and grounding to know how to do so.

In a moral context, we can lose aspects of moral agency and autonomy, as well as lose power and abilities. In my book, *Humanizing Mental Illness*, I show that a form of vulnerability that people with mental illness face is the loss of moral agency.[38] Mental illness impairs agency in both direct and indirect ways. Mental illness symptoms cause losses of capacities such as rationality, emotional sensitivity and regulation, and volition, which directly impair agency. The social isolation and exclusion resulting from mental illness stigma, where people with mental illness are denied the opportunity to engage in moral practices in a community with others, and thus denied the opportunity to develop and exercise agency in relation to others, diminish agency. The world often acts upon us in ways we have no control over; mental illness can be seen as a force in the world that threatens agency, making a person vulnerable to significant losses as a moral agent in both direct and indirect ways.

Mental illness impairs autonomy, too, increasing a person's vulnerability as a moral agent in other ways. In my book, *Mental Patient*, I show that, for some people with mental illness, their illness and the treatment they receive for it can threaten their autonomy.[39] When mental illness and treatment act as external forces that interfere with a person's ability to make choices that are their own and determine what is of value in a way that has not been overly influenced by their illness, they lose autonomy. When mental illness and its treatment reduce a person's opportunity to practice skills related to autonomy—including rational, emotional, and relational processes involved with being a moral agent participating in moral practices in a community with others—the person loses the ability to exercise or even develop autonomy. Mental illness thus makes a person vulnerable to other aspects of being a moral agent, namely the ability to choose and act autonomously.

Other moral losses can occur when a person who might have once been regarded as a moral agent is no longer seen in this way and is consequently precluded from participating in moral activities such as moral address and response. For example, other people may shun a person with cognitive decline and refuse to make moral claims on the person or ask things of the person, so the person lacks the opportunity to try to respond. This can not only diminish their moral agency, but also change their moral identity. When a person lacks the opportunity to participate in moral engagement, they lack important social interactions that can help form who they are, thus stunting their growth as an individual. Moral losses do not only occur as a result of other people precluding a person from moral activity; they can occur whenever a person's situation prevents them from being capable of participating in moral activities, such as severe mental disorder that disrupts a person's ability to understand a situation enough to figure out how to respond appropriately to it.

While Lear's book and my books show how people in specific socio-historical contexts and people who have specific conditions experience ontological vulnerability as epistemic and moral subjects and agents, *all* people are at risk of epistemic and moral losses simply by virtue of living in a world that can act upon them. In other words, some people in certain circumstances can experience ontological vulnerability as epistemic and moral subjects and agents occurrently, when their circumstances cause them to suffer epistemic and/or moral harm; but all people, regardless of circumstances, have the potential to be at risk of suffering this type of harm by virtue of being human, and thus all people experience this ontological vulnerability dispositionally. The vulnerability we have as epistemic and moral subjects and agents is an inherent, universal vulnerability that we all face by virtue of being human.

When Ontological Vulnerability Manifests as Particular Vulnerability

Turner notes that our lives are marked by precarity, insecurity, and uncertainty: always at risk of experiencing harm or other difficulties, without necessarily having sources of security to protect us, at least not reliably. This is because not only are we embodied, en-minded, living under various social structures that govern our lives, and living in the world as epistemic and moral subjects and agents, but we are also situated: we live our lives located in specific places and time periods.[40] Being embodied, en-minded, and situated is a precarious position to be in. Not only are our bodies and minds fragile and potentially subject to conditions that cause us harm or create adversity, our surroundings are not always or necessarily able to protect us, and certainly not reliably; sometimes they themselves cause us harm. How we are situated thus also puts us at risk to harm, making us vulnerable in contingent, context-specific ways.

How we are situated also affects what resources and opportunities we have access to. People who are situated in positions of privilege and power have more resources they can draw upon and more opportunities to exercise their agency and autonomy, which allow them to have more control over their circumstances. This gives them greater ability to prevent or ameliorate harms to which they are susceptible. People who have less privilege and power, on the other hand, have fewer resources to draw upon and fewer opportunities for agency and autonomy, making them more susceptible to harms over which they have little control. Even when people with less privilege and power face the same harms as people with more privilege and power, they are at a greater disadvantage and thus experience greater harm due to their fewer resources.

The nature of the harm and difficulties to which we are potentially subject is dependent, in part, on how we are situated temporally and physically, and what physical and social environments surround us. This makes our vulnerability in some ways particular to us[41]: whatever vulnerabilities we face as an individual are mediated by the physical and social environments in which we live, which can serve to exacerbate or mitigate potential harms depending on the nature of the environment. Thus, while we are all subject to the fragilities associated with being embodied, en-minded, embedded within various social structures, and acting in and experiencing the world as epistemic and moral subjects and agents, the specific ways that these fragilities manifest are particular to us, depending on the specific ways that we are situated physically, temporally, and socially.

While ontological vulnerability is dispositionally universal, having the potential to apply to anyone by virtue of being human, it is occurrently particular, applying only to certain people given their specific circumstances. Although all people have the potential to experience risks as a result of being human, and thus all people have inherent ontological vulnerabilities, some groups of people actually experience these risks based on their particular personal and social circumstances, and thus their potential ontological vulnerability is realized as particular occurrent vulnerability. The Crow faced a loss of meaning because they were subject to dramatically altered circumstances in their way of life when the US government took control of their lands and livelihood; people with mental illness face losses of epistemic and moral agency due to the mental impairments caused by their illness. In these cases, how people are socially and personally situated impacts the way their potential ontological vulnerability as epistemic and moral subjects and agents gets realized as occurrent vulnerability.

Situational Vulnerability

While ontological vulnerability can manifest differently in different people depending on how they are situated, a person's situatedness can give rise to another form of vulnerability, situational vulnerability. While ontological vulnerability is dispositionally universal, having the potential to apply to anyone by virtue of being human, and occurrently particular, manifesting in specific ways depending on how someone is situated, situational vulnerability is both dispositionally and occurrently particular: it does not apply to everyone; it only applies to some people, depending on how they are situated. For example, people of color are vulnerable to racism in a way that White people are not, and people with mental illness are vulnerable to mental illness stigma in a way that those without mental illness are not. Not everyone has the potential to experience situational vulnerability, because it does not arise from the human condition as ontological vulnerability does. Rather, some people experience, and have the potential to experience, situational vulnerability based on a number of context-specific factors including personal, social, economic, historical, and environmental conditions.

Situational vulnerability is thus vulnerability that arises from one's particular circumstances, so that a person suffers from harm or risk of harm rooted in how they are situated.[42] Some groups of people are more vulnerable than others because their social or economic context introduces risks of harm to which other groups of people are not necessarily prone. Some individuals are more vulnerable than others because their personal circumstances put them in an especially precarious position, or because their environment is particularly harmful. Some people are subject to historical processes that affect their way of being more than that of others. Thus, some populations are more vulnerable than others.

Situational vulnerability arises from inequalities between people that grant some people more power and ability than others and that cause harm to some people but not others. Inequalities of power, dependency, capacity, and need all lead some people to have situational vulnerabilities that others do not have.[43] People who have diminished power relative to others are made more vulnerable by that diminishment because they have less resources, opportunities, and capabilities that they can draw upon. People who are dependent on others have greater potential to be subjected to the power of those on whom they are dependent. People who have fewer capacities have fewer internal resources that they can draw upon. And people who have greater need are exposed to more potential harm and thus have greater vulnerability based on that need.

Inequalities that result from injustices also subject some people to situational vulnerabilities that those not subject to injustices do not share. People who are marginalized, exploited, dominated, or otherwise oppressed have diminished power and greater burdens to carry relative to those who commit these injustices or benefit by them. All of these inequalities and injustices put some people at greater risk of harm and thus make them more vulnerable than others.

People who are situationally vulnerable have less power and privilege than people who are situated in ways that do not make them as vulnerable. This translates to having access to fewer resources and opportunities, and less support, which makes it harder for them to access the resources needed to exert some control over their circumstances. Having less power to control their circumstances, and thus less opportunity to mitigate the harms they are susceptible to, they are more vulnerable to more types of harm. In this way, people who are already vulnerable to situational harms are made even *more* vulnerable because they lack the means to protect themselves and improve their circumstances.

Mental illness can both arise from and create situational vulnerabilities. When a person experiences stress due to their living conditions, they easily develop mental disorder symptoms in reaction, which can sometimes turn into a mental illness such as depression, generalized anxiety disorder, posttraumatic stress disorder, or schizophrenia. Many mental disorders are more common in populations that experience greater stress, due to such factors as poverty and urbanicity; this is because living with greater stress can increase a person's risk of developing mental disorder symptoms. For example, in the United States, schizophrenia is more common in people who live in urban areas compared to rural areas, as well as in migrants.[44] Historically, one of the ways that mental illness has been characterized is as a maladaptive response to stress,[45] and this view of mental illness holds true today for at least some experiences of mental illness. People commonly react to stress by exhibiting problems with cognition, affect, volition, and reasoning processes.

In addition, mental illness creates situational vulnerabilities by making people more prone to other vulnerabilities, in part because of the impairments caused by mental illness and its treatment, and in part because of the way mental illness and its treatment situate a person within society. I return to this momentarily.

PATHOGENIC VULNERABILITY

One form of situational vulnerability is pathogenic vulnerability, a vulnerability that arises from negative social conditions such as oppression, abuse, trauma, coercion, prejudice, injustice, or violence.[46] These social conditions cause direct harm by subjecting people to interpersonal or structural harms that can violate people's bodily or mental integrity, agency, and identity; they also cause secondary harms by putting people in positions where they are at greater risk of being subjected to other kinds of harms, such as stigma, prejudice, or other forms of oppression, violence, or injustice. Pathogenic vulnerabilities thus tend to be compounding—exacerbating existing vulnerabilities and putting people at risk for further harms. Pathogenic vulnerability describes situations where the primary harm comes from social conditions rather than from an internal state such as mental illness or an environmental harm such as exposure to pollution. When social structures and systems that are designed to protect us from vulnerability make us vulnerable to other harms, these constitute pathogenic vulnerabilities.

Pathogenic vulnerability sometimes arises from attempts to address vulnerability, as sometimes interventions intended to deal with vulnerability can paradoxically cause or exacerbate that vulnerability or create other situational vulnerabilities.[47] This is because the attempt to administer and manage vulnerability often necessarily leads to forms of social control.[48] Some ways that pathogenic vulnerability can arise are when responses to dependency are distorted, when development of capacities are neglected, or when dependency is exaggerated.[49] For example, mental health treatment sometimes causes pathogenic vulnerabilities in people receiving treatment when it makes people dependent on the mental health system.

Ken Steele describes this pathogenic vulnerability with respect to the way being in the mental health system can make a person dependent on the mental health system: "It's an all-too-common scenario: The loss of self-esteem that accompanies mental illness leads to dependence on medicines, alcohol, doctors, intermittent hospitalizations, clubhouses, halfway houses, SSI [Supplemental Security Income from the US government] . . . round about and back again. There is a dread of independence that makes a person return to the perceived safety of the system time and again."[50] People who become dependent on the system for structure, attention, and getting their needs met have a difficult time leaving the system, sometimes leading people to relapse and need the system again. This can keep people in a state of perpetual harm, especially when the system causes other harms besides dependency, such as loss of freedom, loss of agency and autonomy, and impairments to well-being.

Other ways that pathogenic vulnerability can arise are when interventions are paternalistic or coercive, or when they are abusive, oppressive, marginalizing, or exploitative. Mental health treatments that are coercive, such as by forcing people to take medication or be hospitalized, or oppressive, such as by putting people in restraints or subjecting them to treatments they don't understand (such as electroconvulsive therapy), are examples of other types of pathogenic vulnerabilities. When interventions cause further harms, even in the process of trying to address an original harm, they are pathogenic.

Another way that interventions can create pathogenic vulnerabilities is when they fail to address vulnerability adequately, so they are well intended but insufficiently resourced. Susan Dodds describes the movement of deinstitutionalization as creating pathogenic vulnerabilities in mentally ill people, because it was inadequately resourced and so did not actually meet the needs of the people whom it was supposed to help. When people are unable to get their needs met because they are not given sufficient social resources and support, their vulnerability, rather than being addressed, becomes exacerbated.[51]

A further way that interventions can create pathogenic vulnerabilities is when they are used in situations that do not warrant them. Some vulnerabilities do not need to be addressed through intervention; deafness, for example, can make people vulnerable in a hearing society, but for many Deaf people, interventions are not warranted; accommodations that enable Deaf people to navigate hearing society are more appropriate. Unwarranted interventions such as hearing aids for Deaf people who do not desire such interventions can be experienced as coercive, oppressive, and disrespectful. This creates additional vulnerabilities in people who are already made vulnerable by the way society is structured (for example, as prioritizing hearing over Deaf language and culture).

Pathogenic interventions compound the sense of powerlessness that people feel when they are vulnerable, leading to decreased agency and making a person vulnerable to new and different harms.[52] People who are already vulnerable, whether due to natural vulnerabilities such as impairments or disease, or situational vulnerabilities such as abuse or oppression, already experience decreased power and agency due to their primary vulnerability. When interventions intended to address this vulnerability create further vulnerabilities, this worsens people's already fragile condition and—rather than addressing the harms they face—actually subjects them to further harms.

In order to avoid subjecting people to further (pathogenic) vulnerabilities and to increase a person's agency and power, Catriona Mackenzie argues that interventions to address vulnerability must be autonomy-promoting. By "autonomy-promoting," she means that interventions must help people to achieve autonomous agency, or the ability to determine one's own ends for oneself and the ability to act in ways that help one achieve those ends. Autonomous agency is more robust than basic agency, which is the ability to act on reasons, form intentions, and will oneself to act; autonomous agency involves determining what is of value, setting goals for oneself, and figuring out how to achieve these goals and live out these values.

In a mental illness context, autonomous agency often involves deciding what kind of life one can live and wants to live given their illness and determining what role health and well-being play in that life. Autonomy-promoting interventions often involve guiding people with mental illness to care about their mental and physical well-being, and to develop a health-oriented disposition in which they act in ways that benefit their health and that are in their best interests. Developing a health-oriented disposition is extremely helpful for individuals with mental illness to achieve other ends they choose for themselves and allows them to live the best life possible given their illness. In addition, interventions that promote autonomy and meaning-making must help people with mental illness to develop the epistemic resources to understand the world they live in, and their particular situation, more accurately and more fully, and to be able to navigate these in the course of living their lives. In this way, such interventions can increase the capacity for meaning-making and epistemic agency in general. Furthermore, they must provide people with mental illness the social and material resources necessary for a person to live the kind of life they want, for example fulfilling jobs, safe and stable shelter, and opportunities for positive social interaction.

While Mackenzie focuses on promoting autonomous agency, I would argue that interventions need to promote epistemic agency, or the agency a person has in their capacity as a knower, as well. Epistemic agency includes meaning-making, in which a person makes sense of their experiences or situation by assigning meaning to it, which is another central human capacity. Vulnerable people need to increase their epistemic agency in order to better understand and navigate their situations; epistemic power is crucial for finding ways to cope with adversity. Meaning-making in particular allows a person to assign significance, purpose, and meaning to events, experiences, objects, and people, which is an important aspect of being able to navigate difficult circumstances. In fact, Steve Matthews and Jeanette Kennett argue that meaning-making, or what they call sense-making, is more morally important than the pursuit of truth—and perhaps fundamental to being human.[53] Thus promoting meaning-making should be one of the primary aims of interventions. Interventions must therefore be both autonomy-promoting and epistemic agency–promoting in order to be effective at helping individuals to cope.

In helping a person to gain power, agency, understanding, and a sense of control, autonomy-promoting and epistemic agency–promoting responses help to avoid subjecting people to paternalism and coercive interference.[54] Autonomy-promoting and epistemic agency–promoting responses to vulnerability must address both objective and subjective features of vulnerability. This includes not only the objective harms that people face but also a person's sense of themselves as a (relationally) autonomous agent with meaningful options from which to choose and the capacity to act based on their choices, and as an epistemic agent who can understand and navigate their situation.[55] Interventions that promote autonomous agency and epistemic agency necessarily involve a social component in which social institutions provide meaningful options for action, epistemic resources for understanding and maneuvering one's situation, and the resources, opportunities, and support to be able to comprehend the situation, choose from options, and act on that choice.

Some interventions that promote autonomous agency and epistemic agency include treatment approaches that allow people to make meaningful choices about their treatment, ensuring that they understand their options, and that provide sufficient resources and support for people to enact those choices. Providing interpersonal and institutional care and support that affirms a person's dignity and helps them achieve their self-chosen ends fosters autonomous agency. Changing institutions to provide epistemic resources for people to understand better the experience of mental illness and to be able to assert their needs and make needs-claims more effectively encourages epistemic agency. All interventions that address mental illness by providing the various resources, opportunities, and support needed for resilience should promote autonomous agency and epistemic agency, including all forms of mental health treatment, all interpersonal support, and all institutional changes.

Compounding Vulnerabilities

As we see in the case of pathogenic vulnerability, one feature of vulnerability is that it is often compounding. When people have one significant form of vulnerability, this often creates or exacerbates other vulnerabilities. Compounding vulnerabilities put people in positions where they are subject to further risks of harm.

Compounding vulnerabilities can arise from, and create, either ontological or situational vulnerabilities. Some vulnerabilities—including many natural ontological vulnerabilities—produce situational vulnerabilities by creating the conditions that cause people to be situated in positions of less power. Natural vulnerabilities that people have by virtue of the way their body or mind is—such as those vulnerabilities caused by physical disability, physical illness, mental illness, or mental disability—often put people in positions of diminished social power, creating situational vulnerabilities. For example, consider the way people with mental illness are prone to unemployment, homelessness, and institutionalization.

Some situational vulnerabilities worsen people's natural impairments, subjecting them to greater ontological vulnerability. For example, being poor and homeless can increase people's mental illness symptoms by increasing the stress they have to deal with. Situational vulnerabilities that people have as a result of social conditions that subject them to harm—such as abuse, trauma, violence, or oppression—can lead to physical and mental health problems and various kinds of impairments, subjecting people to ontological vulnerability.

Ontological vulnerabilities can also lead to other ontological vulnerabilities, as when poor mental health leads to physical health problems, such as the way schizophrenia and its treatment cause higher rates of obesity, metabolic syndrome, diabetes, and heart disease. The opposite can also happen when physical illness causes mental health challenges. For example, consider the way having cancer or other long-term illness can cause depression and anxiety or exacerbate other existing mental health challenges.

Situational vulnerabilities can also lead to other situational vulnerabilities. For example, people's gender or race may situate them in a way that subjects them to stigma and prejudice that interfere with their ability to access safe housing or a stable job, consequently contributing to mental health challenges. In fact, having a vulnerability in one area often triggers vulnerabilities in other areas, making it the norm rather than the exception for vulnerabilities to be compounding.

Vulnerabilities tend to be compounding because they are often structurally connected and intertwined. People who have mental illness, who lack safe and stable housing, who are unemployed or underemployed, or who are social outcasts, are likely to have many of these vulnerabilities rather than simply one, because these vulnerabilities are structurally connected to each other. As another example, people who are poor, who live in substandard housing, who rely on informal and not-always-reliable care networks for childcare, and who have low-skill jobs are likely to have several of these vulnerabilities rather than simply one, because these vulnerabilities, too, are structurally connected to each other.[56] Having one significant vulnerability puts a person at risk of having multiple significant vulnerabilities.

The fact that vulnerability tends to be compounding indicates that protecting people from vulnerability often requires a complicated set of practices rather than a single intervention. This is because there is not simply one condition that needs to be addressed, but rather many conditions that need to be addressed in relation to each other because of the way they are interlocking. When people are disadvantaged in one area, this puts them at disadvantage in other areas. And when people lack power in one area, this gives them less power in other areas as well. Addressing disadvantage and powerlessness requires addressing the broader context of disadvantage and powerlessness, looking at the multiple areas where people are lacking concurrently. A complicated set of interventions is needed rather than a single, specific one.

Vulnerabilities Brought About by Mental Illness

Mental illness is a significant vulnerability that compounds other vulnerabilities. People with mental illness are especially vulnerable because their mental illness not only causes mental impairments that have mental and physical ramifications, thus subjecting them to direct harm, but also because their mental illness makes them more vulnerable to various other natural and social harms. Thus, mental illness subjects people both to ontological vulnerability and to situational vulnerability because of the way it positions people.

Mental illness is an ontological vulnerability that leads to other ontological vulnerabilities. People with mental illness are more likely to develop certain physical diseases as a result of many factors. These include the way their mental illness affects their attitudes toward their bodies and their behavior (for example, exercising less and eating more unhealthily), the way mental illness sets constraints on what they can and can't do (for example, making a person too fatigued to exercise), and the consequences of their treatment (for example, medications that cause a person to gain a large amount of weight). People with mental illness are also more likely to develop *other* mental illnesses as a result of the mental illness they already have, a condition known as comorbidity. For example, people may develop an addiction or an eating disorder as a way of coping with another underlying mental disorder, as occurs in self-medication,[57] or as a way of coping with whatever shame they may have in having a mental disorder.[58] People commonly have multiple mental disorder diagnoses because having mental challenges in one area affects mental health in other areas, too.

Mental illness also leads to situational vulnerabilities. People with mental illness are more likely to be subject to stigma and prejudice, to be socially isolated and excluded, to be granted less credibility, to have fewer opportunities to develop and exercise agency, to lack safe and stable housing, to be un- or underemployed, to be undereducated, to be incarcerated, and to need medical treatment. These conditions all cause people significant harms. For example, people who are prevented from adequate social interactions and social relationships risk losing their agency, autonomy, and moral integrity because social interaction is necessary to develop and exercise the epistemic and moral capacities required for agency, autonomy, and moral integrity; and, if they lack social interaction, they lack the ability to develop and exercise these.[59] Mental illness thus decreases agency and autonomy both directly—through impairments brought about by illness—and indirectly—through the social isolation resulting both from the illness itself and from how the illness situates a person in society.

Another example of the way mental illness creates situational vulnerabilities is the way it keeps many people un- or underemployed and undereducated. People who lack employment lack a significant means to engage in meaningful activity to contribute to society, affecting their dignity, self-worth, confidence, and competence.[60] People who lack education lack one of the means to be an informed citizen who understands the way the world works and can navigate their way successfully through it. Being positioned as a mentally ill person in society thus subjects people to a variety of situational vulnerabilities, including epistemic, agential, institutional, and need-based vulnerabilities that interfere with a person's ability to live a good life.

Moreover, the medical vulnerabilities that people experience by virtue of the way mental illness creates further health problems and the social vulnerabilities that people experience by virtue of the way mental illness socially situates people exacerbate each other.[61] If a person has worse physical health because of their mental illness, such as having heart disease or diabetes, they are often subject to further stigma on account of their health condition, especially if the condition itself is stigmatizing, such as obesity. And if a person is unemployed or lacks safe and stable housing, they are more likely to experience physical health conditions because they lack the resources that would allow them to take care of their bodies adequately.[62] Medical and social vulnerabilities thus exacerbate each other, further compounding the effect mental illness has on other vulnerabilities.

In addition to situating people socially in ways that subject them to situational harm, mental illness also positions people clinically in ways that can be harmful. Mental illness treatment positions people as mental patients, a position that subjects people to the potential for further harm. Being a mental patient is being put into a passive role where one is the recipient of care that is directed toward them by clinicians who are tasked with treating them. Both a person's mental illness and their status as mental patients can diminish their epistemic power and authority and often positions them so that they have less credibility, causing them epistemic vulnerabilities and making them prone to various kinds of abuse, violence, and neglect. In interfering with their agency, creating agential vulnerabilities, their illness can make it easier for others to act on their behalf, subjecting them to paternalism and coercion. In addition, being in treatment for illness puts them at the mercy of the medical and mental health professionals who are responsible for their treatment. This jeopardizes their privacy; diminishes their credibility, power, and authority; and puts them at risk of various abuses of power, violence, or neglect, and injustices such as oppression, domination, marginalization, and exploitation.[63] In these ways, mental illness treatment can contribute to many pathogenic vulnerabilities.

Medical and social interventions designed to treat mental illness or address the social problems brought about by mental illness can be pathogenic, producing greater vulnerabilities even in their attempt to address existing vulnerabilities. When medical interventions are coercive, abusive, violent, or neglectful, they subject people to greater harm. When social interventions are coercive, oppressive, marginalizing, exploitative, or otherwise unjust, these also subject people to greater harm. When interventions intended to address mental illness create pathogenic vulnerabilities, they can create situations that are actually worse for people than what they would experience without those interventions.

Having mental illness and being positioned as a mental patient puts a person in a state of greater vulnerability than they would be in if they were not in these conditions, because it subjects them to a range of potential harms that they only have by virtue of how they are positioned. Having mental illness subjects people to compounding vulnerabilities (particular ways that they can be harmed), making them especially vulnerable (increasing their risk of harm). Mental illness is an ontological vulnerability that anyone can experience, but it situates people in a certain way relative to others in society, and, in so doing, it subjects people to other ontological vulnerabilities and to a host of situational vulnerabilities. With all the ways that it subjects people to greater harms, mental illness is thus one of the conditions that create special compounding vulnerabilities that largely come about due to how a person is situated socially.

Conclusion

As we see in Elyn Saks's and Ken Steele's stories, mental illness subjects people to many types of harms. As Steele's story particularly illustrates, mental illness makes people especially vulnerable because it subjects them to many compounding vulnerabilities that stem from mental illness. Mental illness can thus be seen as constituting a significant vulnerability that is worsened by the way it causes or exacerbates other vulnerabilities, subjecting people to many kinds of harms or risk of harm that are structurally connected to each other.

The compounding vulnerabilities of mental illness indicate that addressing these vulnerabilities requires multiple concurrent interventions.

Interventions can include aiding people to develop the inner resources needed to be resilient so they can cope with their challenges effectively, which I explore in chapter 3, and providing external resources, support, and opportunities that enable resilience, which I address in chapters 4–6. As I argue throughout this book, individuals and institutions, as well as society as a whole, all have responsibilities to supply the requisite aid and provisions.

In order to address vulnerabilities adequately, interventions—both those that aid in the development of inner resources and those that provide external resources, support, and opportunities—must promote autonomous agency and epistemic agency. By providing individuals with adequate epistemic, social, and material resources, as well as a range of social, economic, and political opportunities, such interventions give people the tools they need to be able either to change their situation or to adapt to it effectively so they can cope with it. Interventions that promote autonomous agency and epistemic agency can prevent or mitigate the harms to which a person is vulnerable, enabling the person to live a good life despite their illness.

While many vulnerabilities are social problems requiring social interventions, people are often told to deal with their vulnerabilities through personal resilience, by finding ways to change their circumstances or to change themselves to adapt to circumstances that are beyond their control. This individualistic framework suggests that the person who has mental illness is obligated to cope with their mental health challenges themselves and to make opportunities for themselves to live the kind of life they want to live. When we exhort individuals to learn how to be more resilient, we are encouraging them to take charge of their situation themselves and to create the change necessary to cope with it.

This ignores the necessarily social context of mental health response, however. A person can only cope with their mental health challenges with the right kinds of resources, support, and opportunities that allow them to have greater control over their situation. They can only live the kind of life they want when they have the social, material, and epistemic resources to be able to do so, and the social, economic, and political opportunities that enable them to take certain positions in society (for example, to work) and to act in the ways they choose. Even in the context of ontological vulnerabilities that people have by virtue of being human, not by how they are socially situated, coping with such vulnerabilities requires social interventions that enable coping. Resilience is only possible within a social context.

Vulnerabilities of Mental Illness 69

Addressing mental illness so that people with mental illness can live better lives requires providing sufficient resources, opportunities, and support that give people the tools needed to increase their autonomous agency and epistemic agency. In chapters 4–7, I examine some of the external resources, opportunities, and support that vulnerable people need in order to be able to be resilient, which must be provided in an interpersonal context by other individuals and in an institutional context by institutions and systems designed to address people's vulnerabilities. In chapter 3, I examine some of the inner resources that people need in order to be resilient, and I show that these inner resources are developed in a social context where individuals participate in moral and epistemic activities with others. Only in a social context can individuals develop the inner resources they need to be able to cope with their challenges and address their vulnerabilities with resilience.

Chapter 3

Inner Resources

Introduction

For Elyn Saks and Ken Steele, as for everyone, resilience involves many different kinds of actions. Sometimes it involves summoning one's own power to change the situation one is in, and sometimes it involves accepting that one is unable to change the situation and instead must somehow adapt to it. Saks and Steele did both, at different times and in different contexts.

Steele and Saks both used power when they advocated for themselves, asking friends and mental health professionals for support, and working to get their needs met. As a young adult in England, Saks did psychoanalysis several days a week and found it helpful for keeping her psychotic thoughts at bay. Traditionally, psychoanalysis was used on neurotic patients and not thought to be helpful to psychotic patients, but this was not Saks's experience. Knowing that this treatment helped her, she continued to seek out psychoanalysis throughout her life.

She was generally able to find psychoanalysts who were a good fit for her, though she ended a relationship with one psychoanalyst who pushed her too hard and upset her too much. She says of him, "I didn't feel safe with him anymore; he was unpredictable, mercurial, even angry. Some days, I'd walk out of session feeling like I'd been beaten up."[1] She knew what she needed, and she advocated for herself successfully in many areas of her life, wielding power successfully to change her situation through treatment that worked for her.

Saks also used her power in many ways trying to gain occupational success in her life as she became a well-respected law professor. In law school and in her jobs, she learned what she had to do in order to be successful, and she set about doing it. Her determination and willpower were instrumental in helping her to wield power successfully.

Steele found ways to change his situation as well. When he sought out treatment on his own, he used his power to ask for the help he knew he needed. In one hospital, he knew he needed the help of a social worker to progress to moving out of the hospital, and he asked to see a social worker repeatedly until he was successful.[2] This self-advocacy was instrumental in his being able to move into a rehabilitative program outside the hospital.

In other contexts, he used what power he had to improve his situation. Wanting to be able to support himself, he sought out jobs that allowed him to use his skills as a cook,[3] and he found roommates and housing situations that worked for him.[4] When he was ready to live more independently, he sought out an apartment with his name on the lease and successfully acquired a supported housing subsidy to help him pay for it.[5] In these and many other ways, he was able to seek out what he needed to live the life he wanted to live, within the severe constraints his illness put on him. By advocating for himself, he wielded power that allowed him to change aspects of his situation.

Sometimes what Saks and Steele had to do, however, was accept their powerlessness in a given situation and try to adjust to their situation as best they could. Steele had an easier time with this. Throughout much of his adult life, he was in adverse circumstances—whether institutionalized or homeless—over which he had little control. The best he could do was figure out how to survive those circumstances so he could go on with his life. When he was institutionalized, he learned what the formal and informal rules of the institution were and adapted to them. When he was homeless, he learned how to get his needs for food and sleep met. In these cases, he could not improve the situation he was in, but he could learn how to adjust to it in a way that made it more bearable so he could go on with his life.

Living a life that she had more autonomous control over, Saks did not have to adapt in the same ways that Steele did. She, too, had to learn the formal and informal rules of the institutions she found herself in—law school, lawyering, university life—but she at least chose to participate in life within these institutions and so her learning was more out of willingness than out of necessity. Where she had to learn to accept her situation most predominantly was in accepting that she had a mental illness and that she needed to take medication.

For decades, Saks was convinced that she could control her mental states on her own, without the aid of medication, and that she was not *really* sick. After trying and failing many times, where her psychosis got the best of her and she could not control it except by taking antipsychotic medication, she finally learned that the psychosis was out of her control. After decades of trying to go down or off her medication, always winding up severely psychotic, she finally recognized that she had an illness that she could not control, that her willpower and determination were not enough and that she needed to take medication for it. Only after trying and failing many times was she able to see that what she was doing was not working, and that she had to learn from her experience how to deal with it differently, through acceptance. Acceptance of her illness and her need to take medication was very difficult yet necessary for her to be able to manage her illness so she could go on with her life.

Resilience, including the resilience that Steele and Saks showed, is often framed as personal responsibility to deal with a difficult situation, or what an individual should do to respond to their situation. Even though resilience is often framed as individual responsibility, however, it also has a necessarily social context. In chapters 4–6, I show that other individuals and institutions have responsibilities to address people's mental health needs and help people with mental illness be resilient in the face of their illness. In this chapter, I explore the inner resources that an individual needs to draw upon in order to deal with their situation and show that even these inner resources have a social context.

Resilience requires sometimes changing our difficult situation, when we can, and sometimes changing ourselves to be able to adjust to or deal with the situation better.[6] Sometimes it is appropriate to exert power over the situation to help transform it. For example, dealing with loneliness can involve making the effort to interact with others and putting oneself into situations where one has to socialize; dealing with poverty can involve enrolling in school to learn advanced skills that make one more employable at higher wage jobs. In these situations, a person is capable of exerting some power over their circumstances in order to be able to change them.

For this power to work, however, circumstances have to be arranged in such a way as to allow the action to have the desired effect. Interacting with others is only possible within a social context where such interaction is welcomed; this requires that social contexts are not awash in stigma, prejudice, or discrimination that prohibit the necessary kind of interaction. Enrolling in school to learn employable skills is only possible where there is such education available, and where there are jobs available to people who graduate from such a school. Without an employment context that is responsive to a person's need, a person cannot get the kind of job they want. Changing one's situation requires that one has power in the situation, and this requires that circumstances are responsive to the action one performs, so the action produces the desired outcome.

Other times, it is appropriate to change ourselves so that we can adjust to a situation we have no control over. For example, when we have an illness or disability that we cannot help, we might have no choice but to accept that we have the illness or disability and figure out how to adapt to it so we can deal with it. When we are forced to endure difficult circumstances like poverty, migration, or discrimination, we might not have the power to change these circumstances, and the most life-saving thing we can do is learn how to adapt to them to make them more bearable.

Society plays a role in acceptance, too. Acceptance and adaptation are learned through a process of socialization. We learn how to deal with illness, disability, poverty, or migration by seeing how other people deal with them, and we model our actions on theirs. Successfully accepting and adapting also requires that social circumstances are appropriately responsive to our efforts at change, *enabling* us to change as needed.

Being able to wield power in order to change one's situation, or being able to accept circumstances that one cannot control, both require the use of certain inner resources: various skills, virtues, and attitudes that can be expressed and employed in the process of using power and acceptance. Virtues are excellences of character that one develops in order to become a good person, while skills are techniques that one develops in order to become good at doing something. Skills and virtues are both learned through practice and habit, but skills are capacities that can be withheld, while virtues must be exercised and exhibited for a person to be said to possess them.[7] Attitudes are dispositions a person holds that allows them to view events and experiences in a certain way. A variety of skills, virtues, and attitudes are helpful for a person to be able to deal with their situation effectively.

This chapter explores what power and acceptance involve and examines some of the skills, virtues, and attitudes needed to be able to wield power where one has control over a situation and to be able to accept and adapt to circumstances that are beyond one's control. In explaining what these inner resources involve, I analyze the social dimension of these responses to adversity. By no means do I claim to offer an exhaustive list of skills, virtues, and attitudes that are helpful for wielding power or for accepting one's situation; this is merely a representative list to give us an idea of what some of the inner resources required for resilience are and to show how they have a social context.

Power

Power is having the ability and means to affect outcomes through intentional action. It requires both a capacity to act in a way that brings about the desired outcome and an avenue through which one *can* act, or an opening or space where a person can exercise their capacity to act. Power thus involves agency—it is about being able to act, after all—but also requires social circumstances arranged in a way that enables the intentional action to be performed and that is causally set up in such a way that the action will likely have the desired effect. To have power, a person must be able to create desired outcomes through their action.

Power can be wielded either to change one's circumstances or to adapt to circumstances that one cannot change. Resilient actions can involve either. Sometimes resilience involves finding a way to transform the environment or events so that a person can deal with them more easily, while sometimes resilience involves transforming oneself by adapting to the environment or events in ways that help a person adjust to them in productive ways. Both adaptation and changing circumstances require the use of power to create desired outcomes. Which approach a person should take depends on what they have more control over—their circumstances, or themselves.

Power is tied to self-efficacy. Self-efficacy is the belief that one can act successfully to accomplish one's goals or satisfy one's desires, or the perceived capability to act appropriately, given what circumstances call for.[8] Self-efficacy is the sense of power that a person feels in themselves. Recovery from mental illness requires some degree of self-efficacy, where a person feels like they have the power to accomplish at least some of their aims instead of being overcome by their illness. Resilience also requires self-efficacy; a person's belief that they can accomplish their aims supports a person's ability to do so, allowing them to have the power they believe they have to create the change they seek.

A person has to be situated in the right way in their social circumstances to have power over their environment or events. Only when their action is capable of playing a significant causal role in bringing about outcomes does a person have power. And their action can only play a significant causal role when it is one of the most significant factors relevant to the outcome, in comparison with other factors that may be less significant and thus have less power. Having greater privilege enables greater power over one's circumstances, as a person who is situated in advantageous ways can have more causal power in creating desired outcomes and thus have a greater influence on what happens. A person who lacks privilege relative to others, who is situated in disadvantaged ways, has less ability to create desired outcomes and thus less power.

Power, especially when wielded to change one's circumstances, thus necessarily has a social component. How people are situated in relation to their society impacts how much and what kind of power they have. People who are more vulnerable are situated in more disadvantaged ways and have much less power to change their circumstances. People with mental illness, for example, have impairments caused by their illness that constrain their agency and are also subject to stigma that limits what they can do. Increasing a person's power requires changing their social circumstances so they have more advantage, enabling their action to have greater causal effect. When a person with mental illness is socially supported by people having positive attitudes about mental illness rather than stigmatizing attitudes, for example, they are better able to make claims that will be taken seriously and thus better able to negotiate to get their needs met.

Our ability to have power in a situation thus requires that there are openings within the situation for us to exert our power, places where we will be listened to and heard, places where agents and institutions will be responsive in the ways that we need them to be. Through others' responsiveness to our needs, claims, and to our actions, our expression of need and our action can have the power to make change. Others' responsiveness can change our situation, but often they only respond when we make a request, express a need, or act in a way that garners a reaction. Thus, it is imperative that we voice our needs or take action to spur change in our circumstances. Yet, at the same time, our ability to have power requires that others listen to us and are responsive to us.

For instance, when institutions like hospitals have mechanisms to obtain feedback and make changes in response to that feedback from the clients they serve, they provide openings for clients to make their needs known and they empower clients to initiate change. Surveying clients on their experiences in the hospital, both while they are patients in the

Inner Resources 77

hospital and after they are released, are some ways of providing openings for clients to be empowered to initiate change. Such mechanisms are necessary for hospitals to be truly responsive. This responsivity is required for clients to be empowered so that their voices are heard and taken seriously.

Power is social in other ways, as well. We learn how to wield power in a social context where we observe how others use their power. By observing others, we learn what the formal and informal rules are for how to do things, and we learn how to create openings for ourselves and how to overcome obstacles. For example, in a hospital context, a patient can observe how other patients successfully interact with staff to get their needs met and learn from these other patients how to voice their concerns and assert their needs in ways that will be listened to. In an educational context, a student can observe how other students get the attention of the school administration to get their learning needs met and learn what the informal rules are for interacting effectively so that they will be listened to.

In the context of adaptation, we learn from others how to problem-solve and what different possibilities there are for changing ourselves or modifying our environment. In short, we learn how to navigate the world and direct our own action from others. When other people use their power effectively to do the things they want to do and to create the outcomes they want to see, we think of them as role models, people to model ourselves after.

We learn how to wield power *well* in social contexts where others are responsive to us, and we are in turn responsive to them. By participating in shared practices with others, we learn how to engage in those practices well. When others respond to our efforts, we respond back by adjusting our efforts as needed, as the situation calls us to do, in relation to others' response.

Often, changing one's situation requires working with others to enact change. This is especially the case when the type of change that is needed is *social* change. Certain kinds of situations cannot be changed by a single person but can be changed with collective action. Examples include structural harms and injustices like poverty, racism, substandard housing, and underemployment. In these cases, the power that an individual enacts has to be directed in such a way as to combine forces with the actions of others, for only through collective action can structural harms and injustices be rectified and changed.

To be effective at wielding power, we need a range of inner resources: skills, capacities, and virtues that help us take actions in ways that achieve our desired ends. These include autonomy competency skills and problem-solving skills, as well as virtues like courage, confidence, perseverance, and flexibility. I look at the virtues involved later in the chapter. Here I focus on the skills particular to wielding power effectively.

Autonomy Competency Skills

First, we need to have all of the skills of autonomy competency in order to be able to conceptualize what outcomes we desire and how best to achieve them. Trying to change our situation requires first that we set ends, that we create goals for what we want to happen based on our conception of the good. Diana Tietjens Meyers identifies the following skills as important for autonomy competency: introspective skills that help people have self-awareness, imaginative skills that help people envision possibilities, memory skills that can draw on past experience and events, communication skills that can elicit ideas from others, analytical and reasoning skills that allow people to develop and understand reasons, volitional skills that allow people to determine their ends for themselves, and interpersonal skills that enable people to challenge oppressive or harmful social norms.[9] All of these skills are developed over time through practice in which we engage with and learn from others.[10]

Problem-Solving Skills

We need to develop problem-solving abilities that allow us to look at a problem, understand it in all its complexity, and identify possible solutions or responses to the problem. First, a person has to be able to discern clearly what the problem is that they are addressing, and to understand it in its complexity, so that they can consider the right kinds of solutions to it. This requires that they have the epistemic resources to be able to understand and discern within a given context. Being open-minded to different possible solutions is important in order to have more possibilities at one's disposal. The willingness to try new approaches is also valuable, as oftentimes, solving problems involves a trial-and-error approach of trying different techniques until one of them works.

Learning Skills

The capacity to learn continuously, in all kinds of contexts, is helpful here. Learning from one's own previous endeavors and past mistakes what has worked and what hasn't worked is beneficial so a person can apply this knowledge to new situations. For example, in a hospital context a patient might learn from previous interactions that talking to staff in a way that seems to them to be assertive but that comes across as rude, paranoid, or overly emotional is not effective for persuading staff to make changes. Learning from what other people have done in similar situations is also useful. Seeing that other patients have interacted with staff in ways that were not effective for accomplishing their goals, for example, can help a person learn what to avoid doing, whereas seeing what behavior staff responds to favorably can help a patient learn better, more effective ways of interacting. A patient could also ask a staff member what more effective ways of getting their concerns considered might be.

In addition, learning new information or how to use novel technology can also help a person advance their interests. A patient who can learn more about their mental health condition can ask better questions of their psychiatrist and understand better what is expected of them in relation to their illness. A person who can learn how to use new technologies can better access support systems such as those that are available through social media. Learning requires being open to what is new and different and having the courage and willingness to try doing something one has not done before.

CREATIVITY

Creativity allows us to be able to think of different possibilities, and different solutions or responses to problems. It involves bringing something new into being in relation to the constraints imposed by reality. It can be understood as the outcome of a dialectic between what is possible but does not yet exist—what can be imagined or dreamed of—and what limitations shape how what can be imagined gets realized.[11] Creativity is productive activity, where a person produces ideas, in a mental context, or objects, in a physical context, involving sensitivity to the value of what is created.[12] Being able to think creatively allows a person to entertain ideas they might not otherwise have and allows a person to apply what they learn from one situation to a different circumstance. Creativity enhances problem-solving skills.

Creativity is required for adaptation, whether this involves changing oneself to fit one's circumstances, or changing one's environment so it can accommodate one's own limitations.[13] A person needs creativity to think of new possibilities of what changes are required in the self, and how these can be made, or what changes can occur in the environment and how these can occur. Adjusting oneself to circumstances outside of one's control or changing the environment to accommodate personal limitations both involve problem-solving skills where a person has to understand the problem that they are facing in all of its complexity and think of possible solutions.

Acceptance

When a person is faced with difficult circumstances, sometimes it is appropriate to learn to accept the situation. This is especially the case when one does not have control over aspects of the situation; in such cases, acceptance may be the appropriate response. Acceptance involves recognizing one's powerlessness in a situation and not fighting against something one cannot change. Acceptance often requires adjusting to a situation, such as by adapting oneself to it in a way that allows a person to bear it so they can go on with life. Adaptation requires the use of power, as previously mentioned, in transforming oneself or modifying one's environment to better fit one's needs. Before adaptation can occur, however, a person has to accept their situation and be willing to endure it in the best way they can.

Accepting a situation does not mean *liking* a situation. If a person accepts difficult circumstances such as injustice, having few options, or being mentally or physically ill, this does not mean that they *like* or *approve of* their circumstances. It only means that they recognize that acceptance, or forbearance, is the best way of dealing with their situation. Acceptance as forbearance is a normative stance or attitude that a person takes toward their situation, involving calmness and equanimity for the sake of enduring. In some cases, fighting circumstances will cause more pain and frustration without corresponding benefit, leaving acceptance as the best option. Mianna Lotz says, "This understanding of resilience acknowledges that we are sometimes required simply to accommodate and endure conditions that challenge us greatly but which we cannot—perhaps ought not—seek to change or eliminate."[14] Resilience as acceptance has us endure and adjust to difficult situations so that we can deal with them.

Acceptance involves endurance and perseverance: going through or enduring the difficult situation, and persevering and persisting despite its difficulty. Sometimes acceptance requires changing one's expectations, so that what actually occurs more accurately reflects what a person expects. Expecting something that cannot come about can lead to intense disappointment and frustration, whereas expecting something that is more possible, even probable, can lead to peacefulness.

Acceptance is easier if it includes willingness, namely a willingness to go through the difficulty of the situation. We do not have to recognize the situation as positive; we can fully acknowledge its terribleness while maintaining an attitude of willingness to endure that terribleness. Willingness to endure what is bad, painful, difficult, or unjust is a way of dealing with undesirable circumstances that can invite compassion (in the Buddhist framework), ease and joy (in the Zhuangist framework), or tranquility (in the Stoic framework).

EQUANIMITY

One of the ways that people can learn to accept their situation is through equanimity. Equanimity can be understood as even-mindedness, neutrality, or impartiality, and it involves detachment from one's mental states, including thoughts, emotions, feelings of pleasure and pain, and feelings of craving and aversion.[15] Several religious and philosophical traditions advocate adopting equanimity in order to accept one's situation better. For example, in Buddhism, equanimity is one of the four sublime attitudes (along with compassion, loving-kindness, and sympathetic joy),[16] involving the extension of impartiality to all sentient beings.[17] And in the ancient Chinese philosophy of Zhuangism (named after the Chinese philosopher Zhuang Zhou), equanimity is a detachment from emotions, pleasure and pain, and desires and aversions, where these are replaced with an attitude of "ease, joy, curiosity, and playfulness."[18]

The even-mindedness or neutrality of equanimity is a second-order mental state, where a person is aware of first-order mental states like feelings, thoughts, desires, and beliefs and where they are capable of having some control over how they regard their first-order mental states. With epistemic humility, they recognize that their beliefs could be mistaken.[19] They can choose whether they want to hold on to or pursue certain desires or avoid certain aversions. They can decide how to react to their thoughts and feelings, such as by observing them, approving of them, trying to counter them, or sitting with them. In addition, they can reflect on and assess the self-narrative they have of themselves and work on constructing a different self-narrative if they so choose.[20]

The even-mindedness of equanimity allows a person to have control over second-order mental states concerning their circumstances. They can observe their situation, reflect on it and assess it, and decide how to react to it. They can choose to try to change it, if is within their power to do so, or they can choose to accept it. Acceptance is an act that is always in their control, as they always have the choice of whether to endure their situation with perseverance. Through equanimity, a person has control over their reaction to their experience, even if they do not have control over the experience itself. Practices of mindfulness aid in the development of equanimity.

Willingness or Suspension of Judgment

Acceptance is an important dimension of the ancient Greek philosophy of Stoicism. Epictetus distinguishes between the things that are internal to us, namely our mental states and action, and externals, which is everything else, from events in the world to things that happen to our bodies. He advocates that we take control of what we have control over, which is what is internal to us, and accept what we do not have control over, which is everything else. He says, "Seek not that the things which happen should happen as you wish, but wish the things which happen to be as they are, and you will have a tranquil flow of life."[21]

According to Stoicism, in every situation we always have the power to make a certain choice. We can assent to the idea or situation, we can dissent from it, or we can suspend judgment.[22] Dissenting will make us fight against circumstances that we can't control, leading us to frustration. Assenting will give us tranquility or peace of mind. When we cannot assent, we can suspend judgment, recognizing the limits of our understanding and acknowledging that we are not able to make an informed judgment.

People with mental illness often struggle to accept their situation. It can be difficult to accept that one has a mental illness, and that one is supposed to deal with it by following through on treatment recommendations, as it was for Saks. It can also be difficult to accept the particular mental states one has while ill. People who are in despair over their illness often fight against it, wishing that they were not experiencing what they are experiencing. This can make them more miserable as well as exacerbate their mental illness symptoms when they are upset about what they are experiencing. Then, they are not just depressed, for example, but they are also depressed about being depressed. This can turn into a difficult cycle of becoming more miserable at how miserable one feels.

In order to get out of this cycle, a person may need to create some distance between themselves and their mental states. They can do this by developing equanimity, detaching themselves from their thoughts and feelings so that they can observe them without having to act on them or react to them. Then they can make a choice about how they want to react to them, and through this they can gain some control over their mental states. Distancing and detachment, of course, can be difficult for people who lack the motivation, energy, and cognitive focus required for these, such as people with depression, ADHD, or psychosis. Such individuals need more support and resources, especially social supports and resources, that can help them develop this capacity. When individuals cannot change their mental states, they can try to learn to sit with them and observe them without having to do anything about them, which they can learn through intentional practice. Through this distancing, they can reduce the misery caused by their mental states.

CURIOSITY

One way to develop this distancing is through adopting an attitude of curiosity. Curiosity is an intellectual virtue of seeking to understand more than what one already knows. It can be considered an Aristotelian virtue where being curious at the right time, in the right place, and in the right way involves discernment (being curious about the right questions), exactingness (being curious about what is needed, no more and no less), and timeliness (being curious at the appropriate time and not at other times).[23] Two aspects of curiosity include inquiry, or asking questions, and care, being attentive and careful to what is being inquired about and possibly developing interest or commitment to it.[24] Curiosity does not have to be satisfied in order to be worthwhile; the pursuit of inquiry, care, and attention is good in and of itself.[25] Seeking to understand more than what one already knows involves the exercise of autonomy, as one must make choices about what is worthy: what is worth paying attention to and inquiring about.[26]

When a person has a desire to learn more, this can create some distance between themselves and what they are learning about, or between their second-order mental states (of being curious) and their first-order mental states (what they are curious about). Curiosity turns what a person is learning about into an object to be inquired about and understood, an object that can be examined and reflected upon. For example, when a person is curious about how they will deal with a situation, this intellectual seeking creates distance between their second-order mental states (curiosity) and their first-order mental states (misery), allowing them to examine their feelings of misery without being wrapped up in them. Through curiosity, they can achieve equanimity.

Other Inner Resources

Other inner resources that are important both for controlling what one can control and accepting what is outside one's control include virtues of courage, confidence, perseverance, and flexibility.

Courage

Courage is an Aristotelian virtue involving enduring what is fearful for the sake of the noble.[27] Courage is not about being fearless, but about acting well even in the face of fear. Jonathan Lear identifies five aspects of courage, including having a proper orientation to what is shameful and what is fearful, so that one avoids what is shameful and one faces what is fearful; aiming toward nobility; facing up to reality, by fully understanding one's situation and exercising good judgment in relation to it; risking serious loss and enduring suffering; and being rooted in reality and thus not constituting mere false optimism.[28] A person can have courage in situations where they recognize they may not be successful at attaining their goal, as long as the effort of pursuing the goal is still worth doing despite possible lack of success.[29]

Both exhibiting power in changing one's circumstances and accepting circumstances that one cannot change require courage. Discerning whether one has power to change one's situation requires facing reality and understanding one's situation in all its complexity, and making good judgments based on the reality of the situation. What a person chooses to do must be based in reality. Whether they have power to change or whether they must accept their circumstances, they usually must endure suffering in their attempts to change the situation or themselves, in part because situations of adversity themselves cause suffering, and in part because changing circumstances or oneself is hard and often involves overcoming obstacles. They have to face what is difficult or fearful in spite of the suffering involved and do what they know is right, whether this involves actions that try to change the situation or acceptance that it is out of one's control and endurance to deal with it.

Change is difficult, whether the change involves alterations in one's situation or alterations in oneself. Ken Steele notes that people working on recovery often sabotage their recovery because they are so comfortable with the world of illness and dependence that they know, and they are fearful of change. After his voices left him (months after he started taking the antipsychotic Risperdal), he debated whether he wanted to share this improvement with anyone, because he was scared of its implications. He said, "I kept silent about the absence of my voices in part because I thought their disappearance might be temporary. But I also kept the knowledge to myself because I wanted to preserve my options: to return to a world that I knew, one in which I was cared for, or to remain voice free and face the challenges of a new life. The freedom that came with being 'normal' was threatening."[30]

In his decades of living within the mental health system, he had become what he called system-addicted. He knew how to live within the mental health system; he knew how to get hospitalized, how to gain ground privileges, how to survive in halfway houses. He attributes relapses in the throes of recovery at least in part to this comfort with the system. He says, "During the first few months of being well, many people who have suffered from hallucinations quickly get unwell. System-addiction is often the cause."[31]

People with mental illness get overly comfortable not only with how their lives go in the mental health system, but also with how they experience the world while being sick. A person who has been mentally ill for a long time knows how to manage life while being ill but less about how to manage life while being well. Sometimes there is a steep learning curve to getting better. Moreover, wellness can be scary because it is unknown. A person can try things and fail, or have success and not know how to deal with it. When wellness is a new situation, it can be a precarious and fragile position where a person can get hurt and even hurt other people. Wellness can feel too tentative, too unstable, too unreliable, too inconsistent. A person can miss the structure that being part of the mental health system provided or even that their illness provided. When wellness feels unsafe, this can make a person seek out safety in the places that are familiar: being sick or being part of the mental health system.

Steele experienced danger while in the mental health system, too; he certainly suffered many harms as a result of it. However, it became a danger that he learned how to navigate, unlike wellness, which was new and consequently scary. Neither being sick nor being well felt comfortable or safe for him, but what was familiar felt *more* comfortable.

Saks felt danger in the idea of accepting that she had an illness for which she needed medication. She had to face her fears that this meant she was inherently and permanently defective, and that she was not in total control of herself and of her mental states, that there was something else that had control over her. Accepting that she had a mental illness, and that something external to her—medication—was responsible for controlling it, was extremely difficult for her. Her attempts to deal with her psychosis without medication were ways of denying the reality of her situation and not seeing it in its true complexity. It took significant courage for her to face her fears straight on and learn to accept her situation for what it was.

CONFIDENCE

People need confidence and belief in themselves that they can carry out the required action, whether this is the effort involved with trying to change a situation or the effort involved with acceptance and endurance of what cannot be changed. When people believe that they can act in the way they are called to, they are better able to do so, because their confidence gives them motivation and willpower to carry out their effort. Confidence is a middle state between distrusting oneself and arrogance, or thinking too highly of oneself. Confidence leads to improved self-esteem and self-worth.

People with mental illness are more likely to distrust themselves than to be confident, although some mental disorders can lead to arrogance, such as the mania in bipolar disorder. More often, however, a person's experience with illness makes them lose confidence in their competence in many areas of their life, believing themselves to be a failure and believing that they have let other people down. Mental illness frequently diminishes confidence in one's ability to deal with difficulty. Oftentimes, people believe that they cannot endure what is difficult or painful, and this can lead to much anguish and suffering. When a person is prone to suicidal ideation, the belief that one cannot endure what is difficult or painful can lead to beliefs that one must die in order to avoid these. People with mental illness need to build up their confidence in themselves in order to believe that they can endure whatever comes their way.

PERSEVERANCE

Perseverance, or the willingness to keep at one's efforts despite their difficulty, is crucial for both exhibiting power and accepting what one cannot change. In the context of power, perseverance is critical because sometimes it takes a while to be able to solve a problem effectively, and sometimes the roadblocks to change are immense. In the context of acceptance, perseverance is important for a person to be willing to continue to endure what is painful or difficult despite the suffering it involves. For people who are suicidal, this allows a person to keep going with their life and not give up by killing themselves in order to avoid what is difficult to endure.

Perseverance does not require a person to keep up their effort *no matter what*. Putting effort into something that is clearly fruitless is not only a waste of time and energy, but it is a vice. Perseverance requires discerning what a situation calls one to do and what power one has within the situation, and figuring out what efforts are worth putting into it. As a virtue, it requires rational deliberation to determine when and how to employ it. Perseverance is a middle state between giving up on one's efforts and fighting at all costs; it involves putting in the effort required to attain the goal, or putting in the effort that is most appropriate for the pursuit of the goal (even if the goal is unattainable, the pursuit might be worthy).[32]

FLEXIBILITY

Discerning whether they have power to control their situation or whether they should instead accept it also requires some cognitive and emotional flexibility. A person has to be willing to change their course of action should circumstances require it. They have to be able to adjust their emotional and behavioral responses to the particular demands of a situation.

Flexibility is a middle state between being too rigid in one's thoughts, emotions, or behavior to be able to adapt or respond appropriately, and being so open to change that a person loses their core sense of self. Being rigid in their thinking or feeling makes it harder to adjust to circumstances as well as harder to discern and respond to different options. If they get caught up thinking there is only one right way to respond to a situation, they miss out on other possibilities that could be present. If they get stuck in a thought process or emotional reaction, they may fight against their circumstances in unhealthy and unproductive ways. Cognitive and emotional flexibility, on the other hand, allows them to adjust and adapt, and explore different ways of dealing with and responding to situations.

At the same time, flexibility requires maintaining a core sense of self, including core values that guide one's actions, so that one changes in ways that are appropriate to the situation and productive for the person. A person should not be so flexible that they lose their sense of self or violate their values. They need to develop and express values and enhance their sense of self in order to grow as a person. Emotional and cognitive flexibility should be a means for strengthening values and a sense of self rather than diminishing these.

Now let us look in more detail at an additional inner resource needed both to wield power effectively and to accept circumstances that one cannot change: hope. There are several attitudes that could be helpful for a person dealing with adversity, including any of the attitudes that fall under what we call having a "positive attitude," but the one that is perhaps most helpful—and minimally achievable to a person who is in despair—is hope. While positive attitudes can be difficult to maintain when one is in despair, even a person in despair is capable of envisioning possibilities that are different than what currently exists and of desiring these possibilities and acting in ways that try to bring them about.

Hope

Change of any kind—whether we are talking about transformation of a difficult situation or transformation of the self—requires some degree of hope. Discerning whether one can and should exercise power in changing a situation or whether one can and should accept the situation and adjust to or deal with it requires some future-envisioning, in which one recognizes that there are possibilities that could obtain that are different from the current state of affairs. A person has hope when they recognize that there could be *good* outcomes that are possible. Hope is a particularly important resilience factor for people with severe mental illness.[33]

Whether they are able to change their situation or not, people with mental illness need to have some degree of hope in order to be resilient and be able to cope with their situation. Hope in this context involves being open to the possibility that things could be different than they currently are, whether that means the situation could be different or a person's ability to deal with it could be different. Hope also involves a willingness to try actions that could help them make either their situation or their ability to cope different. A person does not need to know what kinds of action they should take in order to have hope; they only need to be open to learning about actions they can try, and be willing to try them. This often involves being open to the suggestions of mental health professionals and other people in their lives, and it often involves educating themselves about their condition and situation.

Hope can involve a stance of curiosity, where a person wonders about different possibilities and ways to try to attain them, in other words they wonder how they will deal with their situation and are open to exploring what that could look like. It also involves openness: a willingness to learn and to try out new ideas. In addition, to have hope in situations where a person feels despair can require epistemic humility, a recognition that their conviction that things cannot get better, or that they are not capable of dealing with their situation, might be wrong. To have hope is to recognize and be open to possibilities, and sometimes this requires admitting that one's beliefs about the world and oneself may be wrong.

On a standard account of hope, hope is a desire that something will happen along with a probability assessment that it may happen.[34] A person is never *certain* about the event they wish for; if they were certain, they would not need hope.[35] However, they do think the event they desire is *possible*; if they did not think it was possible, they would have nothing to hope for.[36] Some philosophers believe hope requires a belief that the desired outcome is *probable*,[37] but I think this is much too strong for hope. Hope only requires a belief in possibility, and it leaves plenty of room for doubt.[38] For people in despair, the goal might be to entertain possibility even in the face of intractable doubt.

Objecting to the standard account, Michael Milona argues that neither desire nor belief is necessary for hope. A person can hope for something without believing in the possibility that it can be realized (basically having the desire for something without belief). They can also hope that something will happen without wanting to want it (in other words, a person's second-order desires might not line up with their first-order desires). Rather than viewing hope as essentially desire or belief, Milona and Margaret Urban Walker both view hope as an emotional stance or affective attitude, or what Walker calls "a recognizable syndrome that it is characterized by certain desires and perceptions, but also by certain forms of attention, expression, feeling, and activity."[39] In other words, hope is an attitude that has cognitive, emotional, and behavioral expressions.

Being able to envision possibilities and form attitudes, emotions, thoughts, and behaviors in relation to them involves what Luc Bovens calls mental imaging. He defines mental imaging as "devotion of mental energy to what it would be like if some projected state of the world were to materialize."[40] Some imaginative capacity is required to have hope; a person must have some ability to perceive the world as different than it currently is, and to be able to form thoughts, emotions, and actions based on hoped for possibilities.

I agree with Milona that full-fledged belief in a future possibility is not necessary, but some kind of belief-like state, such as what Tamar Szabó Gendler calls "aliefs," is. Aliefs are states that are associative, automatic, a-rational, and activated by a person's environment, having representational content, an affective dimension, and corresponding behavior.[41] In order to have hope, a person has to be able to at least *see* that there are possibilities other than what currently exists, and they have to have a certain attitude toward these possibilities involving cognitive, emotional, and behavioral aspects. This attitude need not be endorsed the way a belief must be. In other words, the person must be able to employ their imaginative capacity to envision such possibilities, and they must be able to form an alief, if not a belief, about the possibility happening that affects their cognition, emotion, and behavior. Having the imaginative capacity to envision possibilities, and the ability to be moved by such possibilities, is necessary. I call this requirement a "belief in possibility," even though, strictly speaking, belief is not necessary (alief is sufficient).

When hoping for a desired outcome is not accompanied by a belief in its possibility, having hope can be detrimental. When situations are not in our control, hope for a different situation than the one that exists can feel disempowering as we perceive a gap between what we desire and what seems possible. This can demotivate us, preventing us from taking steps necessary to try to realize our goals, and it can misdirect our agency, leading to disappointment.[42] When belief of possibility is present, however, these issues become less problematic. We do not need to believe that a desired outcome is probable, but we do have to see it as possible. What we should hope for needs to be rooted in reality, attentive to evidence;[43] we need to have some evidential basis for believing in its possibility.

In response to his objection to the standard account of hope, Milona views hope as an emotion or attitude that involves desiring the right kinds of things to happen, with or without belief in its possibility. For Milona, hope is a virtue in the sense that it "is the excellent trait of character that leads us to hope for the right things, in the right way, and at the right time."[44] Hoping for the right things involves having one's priorities straight, valuing the right things, in the right strengths relative to other goods (other things worth hoping for). In order to possess the virtue of hope, a person must have practical wisdom (phronesis) that allows them to understand *why* goods should be prioritized in a certain way, or why a person should value some things over other things and in what ways.[45]

I agree that desiring the right kinds of things to happen is an important aspect of hope, even in the context of viewing hope (as I do) as the ability to envision different, desirable possibilities. Being able to imagine possibilities that are good for a person, that reflect the right kinds of values, is an aspect of hope that is valuable for a person in despair. A person in despair needs to have hope that the future can be good by envisioning possibilities that are positive for the person. This involves having a conception of the good that they can refer to in imagining these possibilities. Possessing some capacity for autonomy is important for being able to envision positive possibilities, and therefore important for having hope.

People who have mental illness often struggle to have hope. Especially when they have been sick for a long time, they may believe that they will never get better, that they will always be sick, and they may despair of feeling like they have no opportunity to get out of this undesired state. To have hope, they have to be able to see that different possibilities could exist, that the future could be different from the present, and they have to be able to see that some of those possibilities could be positive, for example that they could get better, or at least learn to live with their illness in such a way that it does not cause them despair. They have to be able to value the right sorts of things in order to have hope in possibilities that are positive for them.

Hope necessarily has a social aspect. To be able to see different possibilities, people in despair often need other people to help show them what these possibilities could be. Other people thus play an important role in enabling hope.[46] When people with mental illness can see their situation through the eyes of someone else, they might be able to widen their imaginative capacity to see possibilities they would not otherwise see (on their own). Other people can help the person in despair see the evidence for believing that different outcomes are possible by pointing out features of the situation that the person in despair may not be able to see for themselves.

Moreover, other people can help the person in despair envision just what it is they should desire; in other words, other people can help the person desire the right sorts of things. Sometimes people in despair run out of room to imagine positive possibilities and can only imagine negative outcomes, such as death or self-harm. Other people can not only help them to envision different possibilities, but can also help guide them to see positive possible outcomes that are worth valuing. In this way, other people can help a person in despair recover some autonomy, to be able to set ends by determining what is of value.

Other people play a valuable role not only in helping the person in despair see different possibilities for themselves, and the evidence for these, and organize what is of value so they see *positive* possibilities that are worth valuing and desiring, but also in engaging in hopeful actions themselves. Margaret Urban Walker describes the value of other people's hopeful actions: "Hopeful action on one person's part can be gifts of hope to others, who may find it possible because of them to continue living, to trust, and to believe something of value can yet be attained."[47] When other people act in hopeful ways, such as taking actions that assume a sick person will eventually be able to recover, they help provoke hope in those around them.

Hope is an important expression of autonomous agency, where we incorporate the desired outcome into our reasons for acting (and thus our agency), by adopting the desired outcome as an end that serves as a reason for action.[48] It becomes the reason why we have certain thoughts and feelings, and why we plan in certain ways. We justify these thoughts, feelings, and plans based on the attractiveness and probability of the desired outcome. Hope is action-guiding because it helps us direct our attention, energy, and action, and it commits us to a certain course of action. When we hope, we make a commitment to take the actions that seem necessary to realize the desired outcome.[49] We may not know what these actions will be, but we are committed to trying actions that could possibly help.

Hope is action-guiding not only in the way that it can create commitments to certain feelings, thoughts, and plans, and the way it can make us resolve to act a certain way, but also in the way that it opens new possibilities. Being able to envision different possibilities enables action. By envisioning possibilities, a person opens their mind to different outcomes, which they can then use in planning. In other words, they can plan for possibilities they would not plan for if they could not see them. This enables certain kinds of actions that would otherwise be difficult if not impossible.

Hope thus counters the feeling that some people in despair have of being stuck, of having no options; with hope, they can see options. Perceiving different options actually gives people more options because, in replacing the conviction that people in despair sometimes have that there are no options, it removes a common obstacle to agency: a person's own belief in their lack of agency. When people believe they can't do something, they don't do it; when people believe they can do something, or that something is possible for them, they are more likely to try doing what is needed to realize its possibility.

Hope is also action-guiding in that it allows us to visualize different routes that could lead to the desired outcome, making it a genuine possibility.[50] Jack Kwong argues that having a desired outcome only consists of hope when a person can see these different pathways, suggesting that if they cannot see a means for achieving the desired outcome, then they cannot truly have hope.[51] I disagree. Hope can *enable* us to see different pathways, but it does not *require* us to do so in order to be hope. We can believe something is possible without being able to conceptualize how to attain it. By believing in it, however, we can become open to it, which expands our imaginative capacity, enabling us to imagine different ways it can be realized.

Hope does not have to be directed toward an external event, some outcome that exists outside of oneself; it can be directed toward the self. While a person can hope for their circumstances to be different than they are, they can also hope that they can have the courage and perseverance to endure a difficult situation that is outside their control. Knowing what they should hope for—what kinds of possibilities are worth believing in—in cases like this involves discerning the complexity of their situation and facing its reality. When the reality is that they do not have causal control over the outcome of their situation, a person can hope that they will come out on the other side of it and be better for it. Hope can inspire confidence, which can make it easier for a person to be able to deal with challenges because it can make dealing with challenges feel doable. As Aristotle noted, the confidence that hope can induce can also generate courage, which can help a person adjust to or endure change.[52] Hope in one's ability to cope with what one cannot control helps a person be able to gather the inner resources (especially virtues) necessary to be able to endure their situation.

People with mental illness benefit from hope because hope increases their agency and autonomy by providing a means to exercise autonomous agency through the act of hoping and by opening new possibilities for ends to be realized. Hope is thus intrinsically good for people with mental illness. It is also instrumentally good. It gives people more tools for changing their situation by enabling action that they would not otherwise feel capable of doing. It helps people endure difficult situations that they do not have control over so they can get through them and go on with their lives. Hope is important for resilience both by enabling action to be taken to change one's situation and also by helping a person to accept and endure situations that they cannot change.

The Social Context of Skills, Virtues, and Attitudes

We learn what to do and how to be by watching the world around us. What that world looks like—what the people around us do—matters to what we learn. This is especially true for children, who are socialized in the process of growing up and being raised by adults, but it is also true for adults, who are socialized simply by living in a social world. We do not always, *necessarily* learn to do what the people around us do; sometimes we react to what we see by acting in contrary ways, especially when we assess social norms and find them faulty. But we often internalize the norms and behavior of the people around us, and we tend to act in ways that mirror them.

When people around us react to events in certain ways, it teaches us how to react to events, and we tend to adopt the same habits as others. We learn to see the world the way others do, and we learn what is an acceptable reaction from what others do. If the people closest to me—my family, my close friends—are quick to react, I tend to be quick to react. If they are quick to anger, I will tend to react angrily, because I will come to see the world as they do—as something to be angry about—and I will unconsciously adopt their behavior. If they are depressed, I am more likely to be depressed. If they are judgmental of others, I will learn to be judgmental as well. What people around us do matters to what we learn to do.

At the same time, when the people around us have good qualities that can help us to be resilient, we learn to adopt those, too. When other people have faith in my ability to deal with things, it makes it easier for me to have faith in myself that I can deal with things. When other people can see possibilities for myself that I don't see, I can learn how to see myself through the eyes of these others, and they can help me to see those possibilities for myself. When others are hopeful that I can get better, it makes it easier for me to have hope that I can get better, too. We learn attitudes like hope through observing others and internalizing what they share with us.

Not only do we internalize the norms and behaviors of the people around us, but we also learn how to act in relation to our interactions with them. By engaging with others in a shared moral or epistemic community, we learn what appropriate interaction is, how we should understand events and experiences, and how we should respond emotionally and behaviorally. Through interactions with others, we develop skills and virtues: techniques that help us do certain activities well, and excellences of character that help us be better persons.

Moreover, in our relations with others, we come to see certain other people as role models for what we should do, and we consciously or unconsciously model our behavior and attitudes on what they do. We use our social knowledge of what is shameful versus what is noble to help us discern when others are appropriate role models. When other people act well, we try to emulate them (sometimes unconsciously); when other people act poorly, we try to avoid imitating them. We pursue what is noble in relation to what the people around us do.

In addition, in our relations with others, we also gain emotional support that helps bolster our attempts to develop skills, virtues, and attitudes. When others are there for us in important ways, it is easier for us to work on becoming better at certain activities and becoming better persons. The emotional support of others can give us the motivation and willpower needed to act intentionally in certain ways, enabling us to develop the skills, virtues, and attitudes necessary for resilience.

We develop the skills, virtues, and attitudes necessary for resilience through a social context in which a person learns from the people around them how to adopt and exercise these skills, virtues, and attitudes. We learn how to practice autonomy competency, how to problem-solve, how to learn, and how to be creative by observing what other people do, trying out these activities for ourselves, and practicing these skills over time until we become good at them. We learn skills of mindfulness and virtues of equanimity and curiosity in a social context where we observe other people dealing with their situation by enduring it, accepting it with some degree of willingness, and adjusting to it as necessary. In addition, we learn virtues such as courage, confidence, perseverance, and flexibility, as well as attitudes such as hope, by observing others and practicing these in the context of a community that responds to us, by either affirming or criticizing what we are doing, leading us to continue to act well or to change our action to be better. We learn the standards for what counts as being good at these skills and how to achieve these virtues and attitudes by internalizing the norms of our social environment. In this social context, others react to our practices, and how we engage in these practices changes in relation to their reaction through a process of learning.

Conclusion

People with mental illness often feel that they do not have the power to change their circumstances or to cope with their suffering. They also often experience many losses, including a loss of their sense of self, decreased power, diminished meaning, and a lack of hope.[53] Recovery from mental illness requires restoring these.[54] People with mental illness need to strengthen these areas in order to develop the resilience needed to cope with their situation and attain recovery. Interventions to help people with mental illness must promote autonomous agency and epistemic agency, as well as empowerment, meaning, hope, and other inner resources that they can use to draw upon in dealing with their illness.

In their journeys of recovery, Saks and Steele both drew on many inner resources in their efforts to deal with their mental illness resiliently. Exercising autonomy, they discerned what they wanted their lives to look like, given the constraints their illness imposed on them. They were creative problem-solvers who figured out what they needed to do to be able to make their lives go a certain way, and they exerted power in areas where they had some control over circumstances.

At the same time, they recognized the bounds of that power and learned to accept and adjust to circumstances that they did not have control over. In accepting situations that were outside their control—having a mental illness, being hospitalized against their will—they found small places within those situations where they could make choices, and they exercised control in those areas. They adjusted their expectations, and they resolved to endure what they had no choice but to endure.

In discerning where they had power and control and where they did not, and in doing whatever a situation called them to do, they exhibited cognitive and emotional flexibility. They showed courage in making choices where they could, in doing what had to be done, and in choosing to endure what had to be endured. They developed confidence in themselves to be able to do these things.

However hard it was sometimes, they persevered through their difficulties. Both Saks and Steele suffered from depression and suicidal thoughts at times, but they never gave up on themselves. Many times, they also did not let their psychosis rule their lives. However much their psychosis seemed to overtake them, they still managed to find ways to fight it. In their perseverance, they showed tremendous resilience.

Inner resources and good mental health stand in a bidirectional relationship with each other, creating a virtuous circle. When a person has greater mental health, their positive mental states (for example, clear thinking and calm emotional state) strengthen their inner resources. At the same time, having greater inner resources gives people more resilience to face their mental health condition, sometimes enabling them to improve their mental health. Increasing one thus helps to increase the other.

Resilience is often framed as the personal responsibility an individual has to deal with their difficulties themselves. However, as I showed in this chapter, the inner resources that a person has to draw upon in being resilient have a necessarily social context. Resilience is social in other ways as well. The support, resources, and opportunities that people need in order to be able to deal with their difficulties effectively must be provided by individuals and institutions within society. Individuals and institutions have responsibilities to provide people with the tools they need in order to be resilient by providing this support and these resources and opportunities. In chapter 4, I show how individuals provide valuable social support through duties of care, protection, and aid.

Chapter 4

Social Support

Introduction

The person who was most responsible for her mental health, Elyn Saks contended, was herself. She believed that it was her responsibility alone to fight the demons that plagued her and to get well enough to not need medication (a continual goal of hers). While at times she enlisted friends and doctors to help her, she believed for decades that the ultimate source of responsibility for herself was herself.

In fact, for a long time, Saks had a pull-yourself-up-by-your-bootstraps mentality. As she was growing up, her parents taught her that with determination and hard work she could succeed at anything she tried. She believed that this included overcoming her psychosis: if only she worked hard enough, she could have better control over her demons. In part, this came from a deeply held belief that being on medication proved she was sick, and that she would not be sick if she could get off her medication. She says, "Either I was mentally ill or I could have a full and satisfying personal and professional life, but both things could not be equally true; they were mutually exclusive states of being. To admit one was to deny the other. I simply couldn't have it both ways."[1] Because she believed that it was impossible to be sick and have a satisfying life, she tried to deny her illness as long as possible.

For many years, Saks could not accept that she was ill, and she did not see that medication was what helped her be well. In fact, she viewed medication as a crutch, and she believed that needing to rely on crutches was giving in to weakness. She says, about a time when she was extremely ill, "There were plenty of indications that I should do something—talk to somebody, take some kind of pill. I knew that much; I was not, after all, stupid. But pills were bad, drugs were bad. Crutches were bad. If you needed a crutch, that meant you were a cripple. It meant you were not strong enough to manage on your own. It meant you were weak, and worthless."[2]

She believed that other people suffered the same psychological problems that she did, only they were better at managing and—in essence—hiding them. According to her beliefs, "My problem was not that I was crazy; it was that I was weak."[3] But she fought against this; she did not want to be weak and worthless.

She was convinced that her illness was something she could overcome through sheer force of will. She had been raised to believe that with intelligence and hard work, she could achieve anything she set her mind to. "Intelligence, combined with discipline, could overcome any challenge," she thought. But at some point, she had to recognize the limitations of this belief. She continues, "And mostly, that belief had served me well. The problem was, it assumed that the intelligence at hand was fully functional, fully capable—but I'd been told by experts that my brain had serious problems."[4] What she had to learn to recognize was that mental health is necessary for the expression of intelligence, and consequently for problem-solving, willpower, and agency. As long as her mental health was impaired, she could not employ intelligence and discipline successfully to manage all her problems.

Saks found herself judgmental of others who did not fight the power of mental illness, and this led to the loss of friends. Of one friend from a support group who had gone on disability, she says, "Although his intelligence and capability seemed largely intact to me, he'd virtually relinquished any hope of achieving anything further in his life. Instead, he'd gone on disability and worked at various jobs, as he felt the need or desire."[5] In this, she assumed that achieving something worthwhile necessarily involved work or having a career. She continues, "Although I enjoyed the time I spent with him, I found myself increasingly intolerant of his attitude toward his illness and his work. 'I think you've given up,' I said one night at dinner. 'I think you've given in. You're way too comfortable in the role of a mentally ill person.' "[6] This attitude made her lose that friendship.

In the effort to achieve control over her mental states without the aid of what she considered to be a crutch, Saks tried to go off her medications many times. Each time she did this, however, she failed to squelch the psychosis: the psychosis always overcame her, rather than the other way around. After becoming floridly psychotic, her doctors always strongly recommended that she go back on her medication, sometimes at a higher dose, or risk hospitalization. Often, it took a while, and a lot of persuasion on the part of both her doctors and friends, to convince her that taking her medication was the right thing to do.

What helped her learn that she had to take medication to control her illness was the constant encouragement and support of her friends and psychiatrists. Whenever they told her she needed to take medication, she was eventually persuaded by them and would eventually do so. Although she was not always consistent in her actions, she was always willing to listen to her friends and mental health professionals because she trusted them. The concern her friends showed her made her feel like she was worth trying to save, and that it was worth trying everything—including medication—to keep her well. The compassion her psychiatrists exhibited enabled her to listen to them more closely and take seriously their advice.

Eventually she came to recognize that medication was necessary for managing her psychosis so that she could have control over it, rather than it having control over her. With this lesson learned, she was able to reflect critically on her experiences and write an extremely insightful memoir about how her attitudes toward her mental illness, and herself, changed over time. Her understanding of the factors that affected her mental health expanded, and she was able to acknowledge that the quality of her mental health was the result of more than just her own actions.

When Saks learned to accept that her mental illness was a biological problem beyond her control, that she needed to take medication in order to live the kind of life she wanted to live, she came to terms with the fact that dealing with her mental illness was not entirely up to her. Medication played a crucial role, but so did the support and help of others. In her memoir, she identifies many other individuals besides herself as contributing to her ability to overcome her illness. Her memoir is filled with descriptions of meaningful friendships, where friends accepted and valued her in all her complexity, with all her mental health problems, and were there for her repeatedly in times of need. She also identifies many psychiatrists and psychoanalysts who helped her in various ways through the years, in some places crediting her ability to recover in part to them.

It makes sense that Saks would, for a long time, believe that her mental health was entirely her own responsibility. Mental health describes the quality of our mental states, and no one seemingly has more control over our mental states than ourselves. Philosophers since the ancient Greeks have claimed that individuals have responsibility for directing their own mental states, making their mental health up to them. If we do not want the mental states that we have, then it is up to us to change them into what we think they should be.

We can extend this idea to the context of control over our mental health. If we are suffering from mental ailments, then it seems that we need to assess the state of our mind and make changes to overcome these ailments. If we are being irrational, we need to bring reason to bear on our judgments and understanding. If we are being overemotional, we need to let reason calm our emotions so that they may guide us well instead of impulsively. If we are not perceiving reality correctly, we need to bring clearer insight into our understanding so that we can perceive the shared reality that everyone perceives. All of this should be in our control, if we only set our minds to it.

The problem is that the control we need to have over our mental state itself requires that we are mentally healthy enough to *have* this kind of control. This is important to develop not only the willingness to control our mental states but also the self-knowledge to be able to do so. For people who lack insight into their illness, as in psychosis, having this self-knowledge can be very difficult if not impossible, and often requires therapy to develop the requisite insight. We need to be rational enough, and appropriately connected to reality, as well as to have adequate social sensibilities, to be able to discern what kind of mental states we should be having. And we need to have the rationality, emotional regulation, free will, and appropriate interaction with others required to develop and maintain the desired mental states. In other words, having control over our mental states requires that we develop certain mental states that enable this control. To do this, we need a sound mind so that we can have the agency, autonomy, and social sensibility to determine what is of value and develop the commitments we need to exert control. What this means is that we need to have mental health in order to have control over our mental states.

Because poor mental health infringes on our ability to control our mental states, we must improve our mental health in order to develop this control. Improving mental health requires treating mental illness, such as through medication that helps us think and perceive more clearly; learning new coping strategies; being open to other people's perspectives on the nature of reality and the meaning of events; developing insight into why we do what we do what we do and why we think and feel what we do; and learning how to recognize our thoughts and feelings and how to exert some control over them.

Social support is crucial to improving mental health. Through this support, we develop the self-esteem, self-trust, and self-confidence that enable us to take action that we might not otherwise take; it allows us to be courageous and flexible in dealing with our problems. With other people's help, we find ways of handling our difficulties so that they are more bearable. By seeing our problems through the eyes of others, we learn to reconceptualize our problems in ways that make them more manageable. By listening to others' ideas, we consider alternative ways of coping; with others' encouragement, we find the willingness and courage to try different methods. Through interactions with others, we develop our social sensibilities so that we can be receptive to other people's perspectives and learn from others alternative ways of being and doing that we can experiment with and practice in relation to others. Improving mental health requires social support of various kinds.

I begin this chapter by examining the value of social support in promoting resilience, noting that social support can be understood as an interpersonal response to mental health needs. Then, I explain how the responsibility to get vital needs such as mental health met can be seen as an issue of *ethics*, of how people should interact with each other. In the rest of this chapter, I examine interpersonal responsibility for addressing mental illness in order to partially meet people's need for mental health, looking at the duty to protect and the duty to care as ways to understand this responsibility and the way social support can manifest. I look at both consequentialist and deontological grounds for responsibility toward people who are vulnerable, and I show that both approaches highlight important aspects of this kind of responsibility. In particular, a consequentialist approach highlights the importance of capacity in relation to supporting people who are vulnerable, while a deontological approach focuses on the importance of increasing agency as an aim of caring for vulnerable people. Thus I take a pluralist approach that accommodates both kinds of reasons.

The Value of Social Support

A range of studies shows that social support aids mental health, and lack thereof contributes to poor mental health.[7] Social support and health are reciprocal and co-constitutive, as having more of one of these increases the other.[8] Social support aids health both directly and indirectly. In terms of direct effects, social support improves health by encouraging health-related behaviors and increasing a person's self-worth.[9] When other people provide support, their willingness to help and the improved ability to cope that follows from that help increase a person's self-esteem and self-efficacy, giving them more motivation to take care of themselves.[10] Social isolation, in contrast, decreases a person's self-worth, creates loneliness, and allows people to develop unhealthy coping methods to deal with the unhappiness social isolation causes.

Indirectly, social support has "buffering" effects, moderating the impact stressors have so that people can deal with them more easily.[11] Supportive others can also help a person reassess their situation so they can see how to manage (or even avoid) it. For example, dealing with depression is easier when a person has others they can talk to and rely upon for emotional support, decreasing the effects of depression; when a person is socially isolated, on the other hand, they do not have the help of emotional support to buffer the impact of depression, which easily puts them in an escalating cycle of becoming more depressed about being depressed because they are unhappy due to their social isolation and the effects of depression.

Receiving support from people who have gone through similar experiences, such as in a formal support group or through informal networking, has special benefits. Studies show that mutual support between people with mental illness improves treatment adherence, decreases relapse, decreases time spent in hospitals, and makes reintegration into the broader community easier.[12] In addition, it increases self-esteem and quality of life, which can have indirect effects of decreasing mental illness symptoms and reducing the unhappiness and despair that often accompany mental illness. Support from people who have gone through similar experiences provides people with feelings of acceptance, empathy, and belonging. In addition, mutual support has practical effects, including relaying information that helps a person manage their emotional and social problems, introducing new coping methods and providing people with examples of role models who have found ways to manage their illness.

Theorists identify four kinds of interpersonal support that people can receive.[13] Emotional support involves care and concern for the vulnerable person, as well as empathy (which can be understood as a cognitive and affective understanding of another person's experience and perspective based on the imaginative reconstruction of their experience[14]), sympathy or compassion (which can be understood as feeling concern for another person in their suffering, and the motivation to want to alleviate their suffering[15]), and validation. Belonging support connects vulnerable people with a community and provides them with a sense of camaraderie and acceptance. Instrumental support consists of concrete actions that individuals take in the process of trying to help someone, actions such as driving a person to an appointment, helping them to fill a prescription, and making sure they have enough to eat. Informational/appraisal support is information provided to a person so they better understand their condition and situation, such as information about how medications work or information about how to access healthcare services. I would broaden the idea of informational support to include all epistemic support, including offering others conceptual frameworks and providing different perspectives that they can use to better understand their experience and to discern ways of coping. All of these kinds of support play valuable roles in enabling vulnerable people to get their needs met and deal with adversity.

Social support enables personal growth from adversity, and thus resilience, allowing a person to benefit as they learn how to deal with their problems successfully. There are several ways that social support contributes to personal growth. As self-reflection is key to much personal growth, mechanisms that enable the cognitive processing involved with self-reflection help contribute to growth. Some of these mechanisms include disclosing one's condition and situation to others in one's support network; learning about alternative ways to understand one's situation and cope with difficulty; receiving support that helps a person shift their time, energy, and inner resources from being focused on minimizing stress to instead focusing on self-reflection; and observations by supportive others that a person has grown or suggestions about ways that they could grow, leading to self-reflection about what has worked and what they could try doing. When others who care provide their support, they demonstrate that people can be good and helpful, and relied upon when in need, enabling interpersonal growth.[16]

Some areas where a person can grow include external areas, such as having new options available to them (such as changes in career). Internal areas where a person can grow include developing inner resources such as skills and virtues that allow them to deal with their problems more effectively; gaining an appreciation of life (for example, through mindfulness that helps them focus on the present moment); and developing their spirituality. Interpersonal growth occurs when a person is able to improve their relationships with others, as well as when they learn how to interact with others in more positive and fruitful ways.[17] Being able to grow in these areas is a sign of resilience. Social support of all kinds helps foster this growth and resilience.

Social support is aid and encouragement that individuals give to others through interpersonal interactions. The social support that individuals give to reinforce someone's mental health can be understood as an interpersonal (rather than institutional) intervention, or an interpersonal response to mental health needs. Individuals give social support to others when they offer care and concern for what the vulnerable person is going through; when they listen deeply and are present to a person's suffering; when they show empathy, sympathy, compassion, validation, and acceptance; when they help with tasks; when they provide information and the development of epistemic skills and resources needed for understanding and meaning-making; when they help with conceptualizing problems and possible solutions; and when they protect individuals from harm. In the following section, I explain how an interpersonal response to mental health needs—involving caring for someone, helping them, and protecting them—takes an ethical approach to considering responsibility for addressing mental health.

An Ethics Approach to Responsibility for Mental Health

We see through Saks's experience that responsibility for mental health is in part *interpersonal*. How people relate to her impacts the quality of her mental health. When friends are there for her, such as by being willing to listen to her (even when she is muttering psychotically), or by reaching out for help on her behalf, they lessen the negative impact of psychosis and can even play a role in contributing to her psychosis receding. They make the conditions that lead to psychosis, such as stress, more bearable, and they make it possible for her to seek out and accept professional help. When psychoanalysts and psychiatrists fulfill their roles as clinicians responsible for treating her, they help Saks take the steps needed to treat her illness: in prescribing medication and engaging her in talk therapy, they give her crucial tools to help the psychosis subside.

Interpersonal interactions are crucial to mental health and in particular to addressing mental illness. A person can only achieve mental health when other individuals interact with them in certain ways. There are two broad ways that other individuals contribute to mental health. First, individuals further a person's mental health through certain types of noninterference: refraining from contributing to the person's mental health challenges by not engaging in interpersonal activities that cause stress that is difficult to deal with, such as coercion and oppression. Second, individuals further a person's mental health through certain types of assistance: aiding a person in their struggles with mental health challenges by providing or enabling emotional, financial, professional, or other resources that help the person deal with their challenges.

Saks's experiences show the importance of both of these. She describes situations where she experienced coercion during the course of her treatment, such as by being hospitalized involuntarily, forcibly injected with medication, and being put in restraints while hospitalized.[18] She was most opposed to restraints, which made her feel like she couldn't breathe, gave her intense panic and anxiety, and made her act out in response. Instead of helping her, restraints *worsened* her psychosis. In these situations, she shows that individuals can worsen a person's mental health through interference: contributing to mental health challenges by putting a person in a situation of danger and stress.

When her mental health providers *refrained* from contributing to her mental health challenges in this way, on the other hand, by treating her with courtesy and respect, and offering her a genuine choice in her treatment, they actually helped to further her mental health. Saks notes that when psychiatric patients are given choices in their treatment, they fare significantly better. "I had discovered that it was much more effective to be asked what *I'd* like, e.g., 'If you could arrange things your way, what would that look like and how do you think we could help you get there?' "[19] Through noninterference, clinicians can not only avoid contributing to mental health problems but even help them recede by making it easier for a person to accept treatment and to feel supported, lessening the stress and difficulties they face.

People can contribute to, or avoid contributing to, mental health challenges in nonmedical contexts as well. If colleagues had caused her difficulties, for example standing in the way of her tenure or ostracizing her, they would have contributed to her mental health challenges through interference by causing her undue stress that would have triggered her mental health symptoms. As her colleagues were actually supportive, helpful, and friendly, however, they instead avoided contributing to mental health problems and indeed furthered her mental health through noninterference.

Both friends and mental health professionals contributed to her mental health by assisting her in different ways. Mental health providers offered medical and psychological resources, including both medication and therapy, to help her gain mental health. Often this assistance was pivotal in her ability to heal after a psychotic episode. Friends offered emotional resources by seeking out medical help for her when she was in the midst of a psychotic episode, by listening to her when she needed to talk, and by being supportive of her however she chose to deal with her mental health challenges. These different forms of assistance were crucial to Saks's ability to recover from psychosis and to deal with having a mental illness.

We can understand the kind of interpersonal responsibilities that individuals have within a vulnerability framework that looks at the position of those who are vulnerable relative to the position of those who have duties to respond to that vulnerability. In a vulnerability framework, people who have mental illness can be understood as people who are vulnerable to the harms brought on by mental illness, both the direct harms of mental illness itself (its direct effects on the mind, body, behavior, and social engagement) and the indirect, compounding harms that mental illness contributes to through stigma and prejudice; through social, economic, and political power; through dependence; and through difficulty getting one's needs met. Responsibility to respond to those who are vulnerable involves responding to—as well as preventing—the risk of harm and actual harms that people with mental illness experience.

Let us now look at what responsibilities individuals have, whether they are mental health professionals, friends, colleagues, or in other roles, toward those with mental illness. Examining the nature of responsibility in a vulnerability framework helps us to better understand the kinds of interpersonal responsibilities individuals have to address mental illness. In the following two sections, I examine the duty to protect vulnerable individuals put forth by Robert Goodin and the duty to care explicated by Sarah Clark Miller. Both models of responsibility toward the vulnerable have something valuable to offer. Goodin's consequentialist approach highlighting the importance of capacity in determining what we should do and when is an important feature for allocating responsibility, while Miller's deontological/care ethics approach better captures the importance of increasing agency as a motive and aim for supporting vulnerable people. Essentially, I am a pluralist with respect to justifications and hope that whether readers are sensitive to consequentialist, deontological, or care ethics justifications, they will find compelling the general shared argument that individuals have responsibilities to support other individuals who are vulnerable.

Responsibility for Vulnerability

One of the earliest theorists to write about responsibility in the context of vulnerability was Robert Goodin in his 1985 book, *Protecting the Vulnerable*.[20] Goodin takes a consequentialist approach to argue that anyone who is in a position to help someone who is vulnerable to harm has a responsibility to do so, based purely on their capability. Anyone who is in a position to help a person who has mental illness, therefore, would have a responsibility to do so, in whatever way they are able.

Goodin defines vulnerability as susceptibility to harm, when harm is not certain or predetermined but rather possible or probable. When harm is possible or probable, but not certain, there is an opportunity for that person or someone else to intervene so that the harm does not come about. Goodin says, "Vulnerability implies that there is some agent (actual or metaphorical) capable of exercising some effective choice (actual or . . . metaphorical) over whether to cause or to avert the threatened harm."[21] When a person is vulnerable, harm may occur, but it also may not, depending on what that person and others do in relation to the situation.

Vulnerability is a relational concept, where a person depends on someone for something. Two questions must be answered to understand a situation of vulnerability: First, to what is a person vulnerable, meaning what is the mechanism that might cause harm? Second, to whom is a person vulnerable? In this context, vulnerability refers both to the infliction of harm and to the experience of harm that occurs when harm is not prevented. Thus, this question asks: Who has the capacity to inflict harm, and who has the capacity to protect the person from harm?

The answer to the question about to whom one is vulnerable depends on how people are situated with respect to the vulnerable person. The question can be rephrased as: Who is situated in such a way as to be able to harm the person, and who is situated in such a way as to be able to protect them from harm? Vulnerability is thus always object-specific and agent-specific. Goodin says, "One is always vulnerable to particular agents with respect to particular sorts of threats."[22] This is compatible with the understanding of vulnerability as risk of harm discussed earlier. Here Goodin establishes a relationship between the person who suffers risk of harm and others who have the capacity to cause harm or allow harm to occur, and thus have the capacity to do something to protect that person from harm.

In Saks's case, the people who were capable of either inflicting harm on her or protecting her from harm were the people around her with whom she interacted. This included her professors and peers when she was a student, her colleagues and supervisors when she was a law professor, the mental health professionals who treated her, the staff who worked with her in hospital and other treatment settings, her friends and family, and the various other people with whom she came into contact and interacted. All people with whom one interacts are capable of either inflicting harm or protecting one from harm, depending on *how* they interact with the person, that is, the quality of their social engagement.

Vulnerability is tightly connected to responsibility, as vulnerability entails responsibility to protect the vulnerable by preventing harm that one has the capacity to prevent, or by mitigating or compensating for harm that one does not have control over. Goodin regards responsibility as inherently consequentialist, arguing that "'acting responsibly' always consists in acting with due regard for the consequences of one's actions and choices."[23] Responsibility involves being accountable or answerable to others for one's choices and actions; what we are answerable for, he argues, are the outcomes of our choices and actions. Thus, one way to define vulnerability is in terms of the power to produce, prevent, or mitigate harm. Goodin says, "Vulnerability amounts to one person's having the capacity to produce consequences that matter to another. Responsibility amounts to his being accountable for those consequences of his actions and choices."[24]

Goodin specifically argues for a welfare consequentialist view of vulnerability and responsibility, asserting that what matters is the impact of a person's choice and actions on the welfare or interests of the person who is vulnerable.[25] The fact that one *can* protect a person's welfare is a reason why one ought to do so. Goodin says, "If promoting people's welfare is the prime moral imperative, then the mere fact that one person is particularly able to protect another's welfare provides a strong welfare-consequentialistic reason for supposing that he should do so, *ceteris paribus*."[26] If a person does not protect another's welfare when they have the ability to do so, they are not just letting the possibility of harm befall the person who is vulnerable; they are contributing to the harm the person experiences by not intervening in it.

In this consequentialist view, causation is not required for responsibility. Just because one is not responsible for *causing* harm to another does not mean they do not have responsibility to *protect* a person from harm that could befall them. One contributes to harm by letting harm occur when one is able to prevent or mitigate it. Individuals have a responsibility to prevent or mitigate harm when they have the capacity to do so, regardless of whether they have any causal role in the harm coming about.[27]

Vulnerabilities and responsibilities are both relational and relative. Goodin notes that the more control a person has over consequences that impact others' welfare, and the more significant the interests are of the vulnerable person, the more vulnerable a person is to those whose choices impact them. The more that a person's actions impact a vulnerable person, the greater the responsibility the person has to protect the vulnerable person. When a person has less control over what happens to a vulnerable person, on the other hand, they have less responsibility to protect the vulnerable person, because they have diminished capacity to do so.[28]

Anyone who interacts with a person who has mental illness has the ability to affect the person's mental health depending on the quality of their interaction. *How* a person interacts with others creates consequences for the people with whom they interact; it makes a difference if they are friendly, compassionate, wanting to help, informative, having a listening disposition, indifferent, cold, or cruel. People who have relatively closer relationships with a person who has mental illness have greater capacity to either help or harm. They have the capacity to provide emotional, financial, or other kinds of support that can ease the burden of mental illness, such as by making it easier for the person to accept treatment that can help symptoms; by listening and being there for a person; and by being accepting, understanding, and compassionate.

In addition, anyone who interacts with a person who has mental illness also has the capacity to damage the person's mental health by creating especially stressful situations or otherwise harming them such as through stigma, prejudice, marginalization, oppression, or coercion. People who have relatively closer relationships with the person with mental illness have greater capacity to inflict harm if they act in these ways. In social interactions, people are situated with respect to each other in relationships of power and vulnerability, and people who have the capacity to affect the trajectory of someone else's experience have the responsibility to interact with them *well*, in ways that are supportive and helpful.

Goodin situates the responsibility to protect the vulnerable within a larger ethical milieu in which people interact with each other in all kinds of contexts that demand different kinds of moral response. He recognizes that responsibilities to protect vulnerable people can come into conflict with each other and with other types of responsibilities one has. The responsibility a person has to protect a particular vulnerable person depends on what other responsibilities they have, where these must be weighed against each other through moral discernment of what one ought to do. This involves perceiving what a situation calls one to do and comparing this to other situations that also call for action. A person must make moral judgments in deciding which responsibilities to carry out and which responsibilities they must let go or carry out less fully.

Supporting someone who has mental illness is only one responsibility a person has, which must be weighed against other responsibilities in given situations. Some forms of support can only be provided sometimes, when a person is able, given their other responsibilities. Taking the time to listen to a person or making the effort to call the person's mental health professional on their behalf are examples of support of this type. Furthermore, some forms of support are only appropriate within the context of certain roles, such as the medical and psychological support that mental health professionals can provide through their role as clinicians; this support, too, can only be given at some times, relative to other professional duties one has.

Because some forms of support can only be provided sometimes, and not always, Goodin argues that responsibility to protect the vulnerable is an imperfect duty. There are multiple ways of fulfilling the duty because there are multiple moral demands put on us, and we have to determine for ourselves the best way to fulfill the duty and to which moral demands we can and ought to respond. We cannot meet everyone's need and protect everyone's vulnerability, because we do not have infinite capacity to aid. As finite beings, we can only meet the needs of some; we can only prevent or mitigate some but not all harms. Thus, we must discern where our moral response is most pressing and where we could have the greatest impact in protecting people from harm, and act accordingly.

Goodin is wrong, however, to conceive of the responsibility to protect vulnerable people from harm purely as an imperfect duty. There are some aspects of protection that one can practice all the time, making it universalizable in the way that perfect duties are. A person can be intentional about *how* they interact with others all the time, in all of their interactions. Thus, some forms of support can be provided whenever there is an opportunity to interact with the person with mental illness, such as being intentionally warm, compassionate, understanding, and accepting of a person. Being intentional about how one interacts with others is a perfect duty, something one can and must do at all times when the opportunity arises.

The support that individuals receive when others aid them and protect them from harm helps them to act in resilient ways. Aid and protection help a person cope with their difficulties better by lessening the impact of the burden and giving them tools they can use to manage the burden. Acting in supportive ways can give a person the emotional or "moral" support they need to be able to develop and exercise virtues like courage, creativity, and flexibility. It can instill self-esteem and self-worth, providing individuals with more motivation to take care of themselves and learn how to cope with their burden. It makes dealing with difficulties easier and helps a person to grow from their experience, enabling resilience.

It might seem that the responsibility to protect vulnerable people from harm suggests that the ideal is immunization from vulnerability, or the pursuit of invulnerability. However, Goodin rejects this conclusion. He notes that invulnerability is an impossible ideal.[29] Furthermore, vulnerability has some value. Being dependent on others and interdependent with others is desirable in certain circumstances.[30]

As Saks's story illustrates, we are necessarily interdependent with others, requiring social engagement and social relationships in order to develop and exercise agency, autonomy, reasoning capacity, emotional regulation, a perception of the world based on shared reality, and personal identity. As these are all relational qualities, we can only act on reasons, discern what is of value, and exert control over our mental states through interaction with others, where members of a shared moral and epistemic community engage in shared moral and epistemic practices with each other. Through interaction with others, we learn what constitutes reasons that others find intelligible, how to read other people's emotions and how we should react to each other—and situations in general—emotionally, and what is important and of value in relation to a community that sets norms and values. Some degree of dependence and interdependence is necessary, and this makes us necessarily and unavoidably vulnerable. But that does not have to be a bad thing, if people take seriously their responsibility to protect others from harm.

In one way, people are most vulnerable to themselves: to their own actions and choices, and the consequences of these. Because of this, it is reasonable to think that the primary responsibility for protecting a person from harm should be the person themselves. Goodin notes, "It is ordinarily thought that, in such cases, people should bear principal responsibility for protecting themselves."[31] Saks certainly thought this when she thought the ultimate bearer of responsibility for her mental health was herself. She saw herself as causally responsible for not being able to control her psychosis and as having a duty to change her mental states in order to manage the psychosis.

As we have seen, however, this kind of control does not happen in a vacuum. The ability to change our mental states as we desire requires developing our rational capacity, emotional regulation, and valuational capacity in relation to others, by engaging in moral practices with others who recognize us as part of a shared moral community. How we act depends on how others act toward us; we need others to respond to us in the right sorts of ways, such as through support, compassion, understanding, and acceptance; in this way, we are reliant on, and vulnerable to, others. When others interact with us in supportive ways, this makes it easier for us to act in desirable ways, such as (for those of us with mental illness) choosing to engage in treatment, taking medications, showing up and participating in life activities, and interacting appropriately with others.

Because the primary responsibility is thought to lie with the vulnerable person themselves, some may suppose that others do not bear a responsibility to help vulnerable people when they do not help themselves.[32] Goodin argues that this line of thinking is in error, however. While people may play some causal role in creating harm to themselves, they rarely play the only role; other factors are usually relevant, factors over which people do not have control. In any case, once a person reaches a certain threshold of harm, in which case they have no control left over what happens to them, the cause of the harm becomes irrelevant. What matters is that they no longer have any control over the outcome, of the harm that befalls them. At that point, they are vulnerable to the actions of those around them who have the power to help them. Those who have the capacity to help, on the other hand, have a responsibility to do so. People have responsibility to protect the vulnerable regardless of whether the vulnerable contributed to their own experience of harm, just because they have the capacity to do so.[33]

For example, Saks caused herself harm when she refused to take her medication, even though she needed it, because of mistaken beliefs about the role the medication played in her life. Through her own intentionally willed actions, she set herself up for experiencing bad outcomes, and thus she was at least partly causally responsible for what happened to her. Nevertheless, the people around her should not have just let her continue to pursue her own harm; they should have tried to help her, as her close friends did, because they had the capacity to do so and because they had a duty to, and in fact did, care. Moreover, her unwillingness to take medication could be seen as a symptom of her illness over which she had no control and thus ultimately was *not* responsible for. When people contribute to their own harm, their actions are only one part of a complicated causal chain; isolating them as the sole or primary cause of the outcome is not usually sensical.

Critics might worry that the duty to protect even in cases where vulnerable people contributed to their own harm would lead people to overrely on others to get themselves out of a mess of their own making. Goodin concedes this is a possibility and recommends that we should encourage vulnerable people to avoid getting themselves into such messes.[34] Education can help people learn how to avoid causing themselves harm, while persuasion and incentives can motivate people to act in their best interests. In the context of mental illness, this points to an important role that mental health professionals play in helping people with mental illness to learn how to take care of themselves, and to give people with mental illness reasons and incentives that make them want to take care of themselves.[35]

Critics might also object that it is too much of a moral burden to place the responsibility for protecting vulnerable people from harm on those who happen to have the capacity to do so, that they do not deserve this moral burden.[36] Helping people in this context should be considered supererogatory but not obligatory: a morally praiseworthy act, but not morally required. Goodin counters that desert is irrelevant to whether someone has certain obligations or not. He argues, "Duties and responsibilities are not necessarily (or even characteristically) things that you deserve. More often than not, they are things that just happen to you."[37]

Responsibilities are imposed on us by circumstances beyond our control, and sometimes beyond any particular person's control. Situations just arise, through a confluence of causal factors, calling on us to respond in some way. As moral agents, we are obligated to respond to those circumstances as best as we can, and when the circumstances are such that we are in a position to aid people who are vulnerable to harm, the situation calls on us to do so. While some critics might worry that a consequentialist approach to responsibility is overly burdensome, I believe that consequentialist reasons for acting simply reflect a fact about how we do and ought to interact with others: responding to claims they make as best as we can given our circumstances. In the context of mental illness, we are called upon to interact in intentionally supportive ways whenever we find ourselves interacting with someone who has mental illness.

Another criticism often lodged against consequentialist approaches to morality and responsibility is that they can fail to respect personhood, agency, and dignity when they allow the sacrifice of a person's dignity or agency for the sake of a morally desirable outcome. Protecting the vulnerable can have unintended consequences of making some people more vulnerable in the process of trying to protect others. Consequentialism, therefore, cannot be the only guiding principle to act on in addressing vulnerability. Deontological principles of respecting all relevant agents' dignity and agency must apply as well. In the next section, I examine Miller's deontological/care ethics theory of how and why we should protect the vulnerable, which explicitly supports the dignity and agency of all vulnerable people.

While Goodin's theory of responsibility for vulnerability seems to apply primarily to individuals in an interpersonal context, it can also be extended to an institutional context. Goodin argues that individuals generally have primary duties to protect the vulnerable, based on such things as relationships (such as parents to children) or contracts (such as employers to employees). But in circumstances where individuals are unable or unwilling to discharge these primary responsibilities, secondary responsibilities must be assigned instead. Those who have secondary responsibilities to protect the vulnerable are those that have the greatest capacity to do so. Goodin argues that in general, this is the state.[38] I address institutional responsibilities in greater detail in chapter 6.

What I have done here is show how responsibility to protect people from vulnerability falls on all of us as individuals, whenever we find ourselves in a situation that calls upon us to respond to the plight of others. Responsibility to protect people from the harms of mental illness is a responsibility we all share whenever we are interacting with people who have or may have mental illness. Some people might not be convinced that capacity alone is what grounds responsibility toward the vulnerable, however. They might believe that responsibility should be grounded on a moral fact about the person, such as the person's inherent dignity and worth as an autonomous agent. Reciprocity of need and agency based on dignity and worth can also ground responsibility. In the next section, I show how this duty to protect can also be understood and argued for in terms of a combination of care ethics and Kantian ethics.

The Duty to Care

The responsibility to protect the vulnerable can also be understood in terms of a duty to care. Sarah Clark Miller grounds the duty to care in the Kantian duty of beneficence.[39] This duty is both universalizable and respects other people as ends in themselves. We have a duty of beneficence because we cannot will a world in which no one helps others; everyone is interdependent on others to get their needs met and thus to be able to exercise their (autonomous) agency as a human being, where agency is understood as the ability to set ends for oneself and to pursue those ends through action, or the ability to act on reasons based on one's values.[40] Sometimes I am needy of others' help, and sometimes others are needy and I am able to help them. In respecting our own dignity as human beings, as well as the dignity of others, we can only will a world in which people help those in need, so that our own needs get met, and others' needs get met, too. We must will to help others in order to ensure our own continued survival.[41]

Agency necessarily has a social dimension: in order to develop and exercise my agency, I am dependent on others to aid me in these processes, to help me to learn how to be an agent and to give me opportunities to exercise my agency through interactions with others. I thus need others to help me in the exercise of my agency. Similarly, other people need help to develop and exercise their agency. When I am in a position where I am capable of helping others develop and exercise their agency, I have a duty to do so, just as they have a duty to help me when they can. The needs of agency thus ground a reciprocity of assistance in helping to meet those needs.

Agency has a social dimension in another way, too: it is not just that exercising agency requires a moral community in which to engage in moral practices with others, but exercising agency also requires that certain basic needs are met, which must be accomplished through interdependent relations. I have certain needs that must be met to be able to exercise my agency; if I am starving, for example, my agency will be severely compromised. As an interdependent creature, I need others to help me get my needs met. According to the duty of beneficence, others are obligated to help me get my needs met so that I may exercise my agency; consistency demands that I have the same obligation to help others get *their* needs met so they can exercise *their* agency. We are interdependent on each other for getting our basic needs met in order to maintain our agency.[42] The needs of agency thus also ground a reciprocity of assistance in helping to get each other's basic needs met.

In the context of mental illness, this means that we are obligated to help people with mental illness get their needs for agency met, both through providing a place for them to develop and exercise their agency, and through assisting them in getting their basic needs met. What this means is that we must invite people with mental illness into our moral and epistemic communities and interact with them as we engage in shared moral and epistemic practices, not as a one-off deal but in an ongoing way. We must be committed to ongoing, intentional interaction with people with mental illness so they may exercise their agency. The friends and colleagues who interacted with Saks in everyday life, and the mental health professionals who treated Saks over the long term, all showed commitment to engaging in ongoing, intentional interaction with her in ways that fostered her agency.

We are also obligated to help people with mental illness get their basic needs for such things as food, shelter, and healthcare met so that they may have the basic requirements that enable agency. In Saks's case, this meant ensuring that Saks had food and water, a place to live, and healthcare access. While these were not a concern for her, they were much more of a concern for Ken Steele, who sometimes lacked food, shelter, and healthcare access, particularly when he was homeless. It was paramount that people who came into contact with Steele helped him to acquire the basic requirements that enable agency. This occurred occasionally when psychiatrists reached out to him, as a homeless person, to help him connect with mental health treatment, or when the mental health system helped him find a job and a place to live. As Steele's example shows, helping people get their basic needs met is more the job of institutional structures than of individuals, but individuals do play a role in enabling institutions to do this.

Care involves many different types of actions. In some contexts, care involves giving emotional support, and providing empathy, sympathy, compassion, validation, and acceptance. Care as emotional support often requires listening to a person's story deeply and simply being present to their suffering. In other contexts, care involves performing tasks of helping, such as helping to fulfill a person's medication prescription, driving them to an appointment, or taking them grocery shopping.

Care can also involve providing epistemic resources so that a person can understand their situation better and figure out how to cope. In this context, providing information, conceptual frameworks, and suggestions can be helpful; providing opportunities for meaning-making can also be crucial. Susan Brison notes that recovery from trauma often requires telling one's story to an empathetic listener.[43] As an aspect of care, listening to a person's narrative of their own experience can be critical.

In a professional context, care can involve carrying out one's professional duties with empathy and compassion. Clinical empathy involves imaginatively reconstructing the patient's experience in order to have a cognitive and affective understanding of the patient's experience, seeing it from their own point of view.[44] Clinical compassion is an attitude of helpfulness, or a benevolent response to suffering,[45] where a clinician recognizes the suffering of the patient, possibly even feels distress on their behalf, and is motivated to respond to it.[46] When clinicians empathize with and feel compassion for their patients, this improves the quality of care they give, enhances patient response to treatment recommendations, and makes patients feel cared for.[47] In a professional context, care can involve carrying out one's professional duties with empathy (which can be understood as a cognitive and affective understanding of another person's experience and perspective based on the imaginative reconstruction of their experience[48]), and compassion (which can be understood as feeling concern for another person in their suffering, and the motivation to want to alleviate their suffering[49]).

The duty to care is grounded in autonomous agency. Kant specifically grounds the duty of beneficence, which is the basis for the duty to care, in rational, autonomous agency. According to Kant, as rational and autonomous agents, we are able to set ends for ourselves, deciding for ourselves what is of value and what goals we should strive for. This end-setting capacity is what distinguishes humans from other animals. Miller expands Kant's notion of agency to include emotional and relational aspects as well: acting in the world and setting ends involves not only reasoning capacities, but also social and emotional capacities.[50] Miller thus grounds the duty of caring in a more complex notion of agency that includes rational, emotional, and relational aspects.

One of the ends that we can set for ourselves is the adoption of *other people's* ends. Miller describes this as a "unique moral power":[51] the ability to not only express our own self-determination through the adoption of our own ends, but also to help others pursue their own self-determination by adopting their ends for ourselves. Through adopting others' ends as our own, we exercise our moral agency by participating in moral practices of aiding others to further their own aims. We treat the others whose ends we adopt as members of a shared moral community who participate in shared moral practices, which here we can understand as the pursuit of one's chosen ends.

Helping others pursue their own ends is a way of recognizing and respecting their agency and consequently their dignity as human beings. When we help others achieve their own ends, we are helping them to exercise their autonomous agency, aiding them in the process of trying to secure their ends. In this way, we acknowledge their status as moral agents. Thus, while we exercise our own moral agency through adopting others' ends as our own, we also enable others to exercise theirs.

What this means in the context of mental illness is that we ought to find ways to help people with mental illness determine and pursue their own chosen ends. When mental health professionals encouraged Saks to continue her education and to pursue her career as a law professor, they helped her pursue her self-chosen ends. When social workers helped Steele find a job and a place to live, they helped him pursue his self-chosen ends. When friends were supportive of Saks by listening and being there for her, they helped her pursue her self-chosen ends, too.

Helping others pursue their own ends is a mode of caring. Insofar as we have a duty to help others in need, we have a duty to care for them. Miller says, "The duty to care obliges others to respond to individuals' fundamental needs so that those individuals can once again determine and seek their own subjective ends (an ability many regard as being characteristically human)."[52] Certainly the duty of care does not require the carer to adopt *all* of the ends of the person being cared for, but it does entail that the carer discern which ends should be adopted by prioritizing the ends that have the most moral weight and urgency, such as ends necessary for survival and agency.

There is a certain form of reciprocity in the duty to care, though the duty is not strictly reciprocal. We need other people's help in order to meet our basic needs so that we may exercise our agency, and others need our help in order to meet *their* needs so they may exercise *their* agency. This reciprocity does not need to be, and usually is not, an equal exchange between two parties, but rather a looser relationship where sometimes a person is needy, and sometimes they are in a position to help others in need.[53] Miller calls this relationship of need and dependency reciprocity-in-connection.[54]

Sometimes this relationship is lopsided: some people have significant, chronic needs and are not in a position to be able to give much help to others, while some people have lesser needs and much greater capacity to help others. This lopsidedness is perfectly compatible with the way the duty to care gets expressed: as vulnerable, needy, finite individuals, people have the needs they have, and when they have the capacity to help others in their vulnerability, neediness, and finiteness, they have the obligation to do so. The duty gets expressed when there is need and when there is someone in a position to help, whenever a person happens to be in either position.

On the surface, the duty to care appears to be lopsided when we examine the life of someone like Steele. For much of his adult life, Steele was very needy and dependent on others, and the mental health system, to get his needs met. However, when he had the opportunity, Steele also found ways to give to others and help others meet *their* needs. He helped found a voting registration drive for people with mental illness to acquire the ability to express their voice through voting; he edited a publication that gave voice to the concerns and needs of people with mental illness; and, through talks and interviews, he provided advice and counsel to friends, family members, and people with mental illness themselves. Steele was not able to engage in most of these activities while in the throes of his illness, but he did engage in them when he acquired the capacity to do so. People who are particularly needy and dependent on others often find ways to give to others and help meet other people's needs when they have the capacity to do so.

According to Miller, the duty to care, like the Kantian duty of beneficence, is an imperfect duty, meaning that we have discretion in choosing which actions to take up in order to fulfill the duty.[55] Miller notes that there are multiple varieties of caring and multiple actions that one can perform to fulfill this duty; a person has discretion in choosing which actions to perform.[56] Individuals do not need to feel a certain kind of love and affection toward the people they care for. The duty to care provides practical love to another person, which is not a particular kind of emotion but rather a way of acting that is not indifferent but rather responsive.[57]

However, I would argue that, just as Goodin's consequentialist responsibility to protect the vulnerable has a perfect duty component, namely that a person ought always to interact in intentionally supportive ways whenever they have the opportunity to do so, the duty to care similarly has a perfect duty component. One of the aspects of caring has to do with how a person interacts with others. A person always has the obligation to interact in supportive ways; there is discretion in what specific actions this involves, but there is no discretion in whether a person ought to interact intentionally. The duty to care, like the responsibility to protect the vulnerable, has a perfect duty component in requiring us always to act intentionally in ways that are supportive to people with mental illness.

In addition to having a perfect duty component that the more general duty of beneficence lacks, the duty of care is also stronger than a more general duty of beneficence. While beneficence involves helping people in order to benefit them in some way, care involves meeting people's needs so they can achieve ultimate ends of being human such as survival and autonomous agency. The duty of care can be understood as one specific form, albeit a very special one, of the more general duty of beneficence.

There are constraints on the degree of self-sacrifice that a person is expected to give in carrying out the duty of care. In caring for others, a person must still be able to pursue their own self-determined ends, life projects, and happiness. They still have the Kantian duty to promote their own talents and abilities and must have the means to do so even in the process of giving care.[58] Like Goodin, Miller recognizes that the duty to care is one of many obligations a person has, and they must balance this responsibility with their other responsibilities.

Miller acknowledges that there are tensions inherent in competing needs. She notes, "Human finitude entails a world in which we encounter more need than we can meet."[59] In fulfilling our duty to care, we must discern where the greatest needs are, how best these needs will be served, what our own contributions to helping others can be, and what relationships we have that make some demands for help more pressing than others. We must use moral judgment to determine where we should fulfill our duty to care and how we can best accomplish this. We must acknowledge that we cannot do everything that needs to be done, but be satisfied that we are contributing to helping those in need when we are doing our best given the very real constraints we have on what we can do.

While the responsibility to protect the vulnerable can sometimes be paternalistic, depending on the kind of action one performs, the duty to care is nonpaternalistic: it involves helping another person to decide for themselves what ends to pursue, and to help them pursue their own

Social Support 123

self-determined ends. Caring does not involve determining oneself what ends the person being cared for should have, or deciding for the person how they should try to achieve their ends. In a caring relationship, the person being cared for should define and express their self-chosen ends themselves, and the person caring for them should respect and honor that choice, helping the person being cared for to be able to accomplish the ends they have set for themselves.[60]

In the context of mental illness, this means that people with mental illness must have the right to decide for themselves what is of value and what is worth pursuing beyond the basic needs that are required for basic agency. Moreover, they must be helped in pursuing *these* ends, not the ends that caretakers, mental health professionals, and other people in the person's life might choose. The duty to care is necessarily autonomy-promoting and thus can avoid causing pathogenic vulnerabilities that sometimes occur as a result of paternalistic interventions.

It is important to dignify care: to care in a way that maintains the dignity of the person being cared for by respecting them as ends in themselves. This requires us to respect their ability to set ends for themselves by honoring the ends they do set for themselves.[61] People have dignity in the sense that they have inherent and unconditional worth, not as rational autonomous beings, as Immanuel Kant would have it,[62] but rather as beings that have interests. Paul Taylor identifies beings that have inherent worth and interests of their own as beings that have a good of their own, independently of anyone's valuation of it, based at least in part on having biological functions aiming at survival, flourishing, and propagation of the species.[63] Such beings have well-being that can be benefited or harmed by particular actions; because they have inherent worth, their interests must be respected. Agents should have a disposition to benefit rather than harm them. Beings with biological functions and aims, including human beings, as well as animals and plants, have interests in flourishing; there is a moral imperative to respect these interests as the "biologically goal-directed activity of natural entities."[64] Dignifying care involves respecting people's inherent and unconditional worth as beings that have interests in flourishing.

While the ability to set ends for oneself is not essential to have dignity (rather, having an interest in flourishing is), it is nonetheless one aspect of dignity that is of central value for people who have this capacity. Insofar as people are able to set ends for themselves, then, these ends must be respected for care to be dignifying. Autonomy-promoting interventions, as discussed in chapter 2, help to maintain the dignity of the person who receives the intervention; when people act in supportive ways, they maintain the dignity of the person they are supporting when they respect the ends and choices the person makes. Care that is dignifying promotes resilience because, by enabling agency and autonomy, it gives individuals the support and tools they need to be able to develop inner resources and employ these effectively.

Care that is not dignifying, such as interventions that impose one's will on a person, can cause additional harm to people who are already vulnerable, further damaging their agency. Interventions that are intended to meet people's needs can *appear* to be caring, but if they do not respect individuals' self-chosen ends, they are not *in fact, properly* caring, because they do not promote individuals' agency but rather set it back further. Care that is not dignifying, that does not promote autonomous agency, does not help individuals develop or exercise the inner resources they need to be resilient.

Sometimes people are not able to set autonomous ends for themselves, such as when a person's mental illness makes them want to self-injure or even kill themselves. In these cases, it is important for the carer to understand the person's point of view as much as possible and help guide the person to choose ends that further their well-being. Mental health professionals as well as friends and family members play an important role in helping people to develop care for themselves, to learn *how* to care for themselves, and to choose better ends for themselves. Such care should not be coercive—imposing ends on the person—but rather guiding and supporting them to choose ends that are in their best interests.

Care that is dignifying involves many specific practices. With moral perception and moral judgment, one recognizes what is morally salient (when someone is in need, and how) and is attentive to the situation and sensitive to the context. With emotional attunement to the person in need, one is sensitive to the emotional context and affectionate where affection is called for (but not when it is not). Awareness of power relations requires that one examines and is aware of one's beliefs, judgments, and attitudes, particularly to the person they are caring for and to the states of neediness, vulnerability, and dependence in general. A caring individual must cultivate the self-determination of the person who is being cared for. Caring also requires recognizing the way the person being cared for is situated, as well as the self doing the caring, and appreciating the various differences in people who are being cared for.[65]

In supporting people with mental illness, there are limits to what a person can and should do, especially for people who are themselves vulnerable, such as children of parents who have mental illness. Individuals need to be self-aware of their limitations and ensure that in offering care to others, they also prioritize their self-care, so in trying to meet other people's needs, they do not sacrifice their own needs in the process. In the context of providing dignifying care, this means that individuals need to let themselves have the time, energy, and resources to pursue their self-chosen ends even as they help the people they support to pursue those people's own ends. In other words, while supporting others can involve *some* sacrifice, individuals offering support must not sacrifice at least the most important of their self-chosen ends and needs. For children of mentally ill parents of any age, they must not sacrifice their own needs for personal growth and development, including their needs for education, work, and a social life, even as they devote some of their time, energy, and resources toward attending to their parents.

Grounding the duty of care in the Kantian duty of beneficence is an ingenious way of understanding what care involves—aiding others in their need—and why it is important: as a way to secure one's own and others' autonomous agency (the ability to set and pursue ends of one's own choosing), which is of fundamental importance for humans. The human condition of being finite, vulnerable, and needy makes securing agency sometimes challenging, as many obstacles can get in the way of our ability to set and pursue ends. Only with the help of others can we overcome many of these obstacles, and only by helping others can others overcome some of their own obstacles. Exercising agency is a necessarily interdependent process of helping others in their need and being helped when one is in need themselves.

Miller's theory of the duty to care is a helpful way to understand the responsibility that individuals have toward others in the interpersonal sphere. It does not automatically provide a way to understand the responsibility that *institutions* have toward those in need, but its prescriptions can apply to the individuals who work in these institutions in terms of how they should interact with those they are caring for. For instance, social workers have a duty to provide dignifying care that is appropriately responsive and respectful of people's self-chosen ends without having specific emotional content. It is not clear if institutions have a duty to care, how such a duty would be grounded at an institutional level, or what this duty looks like institutionally, but people working within certain institutions surely have this duty toward the people whom they are helping through their role in the institution.

Conclusion

As we see from Saks's experience, support from others—both the social support from friends and the professional support from mental health professionals—is extremely valuable to people with mental illness. It mattered tremendously to her welfare that her friends listened to her and took care of her, that her colleagues were warm and supportive, and that her psychiatrists/psychoanalysts provided effective, warm, and professional treatment.

The consequentialist responsibility to protect the vulnerable and the Kantian/care ethics duty to care are two important ways to conceptualize the responsibility we have toward people who are made vulnerable by mental illness. While each grounds responsibility in a different way, both theories promote the importance of autonomous agency and the way such agency is necessarily relational and social. Both conceptualize human beings as beings who are necessarily dependent on, and interdependent with, each other to realize our autonomous agency. Because we are interdependent on each other to get our agency needs met, we must rely on the care and concern of others, and their ability to play a role in both protecting us from harm and helping to promote our autonomy.

Both the responsibility to protect the vulnerable and the duty to care focus on the responsibilities that individuals have qua individuals to respond to the needs of the vulnerable. Thus, both kinds of duties are *interpersonal* responsibilities best understood in an ethics framework, namely consequentialism for the former and Kantianism and care ethics for the latter. In the context of mental illness, they show what kinds of responsibilities individuals have to respond to the actual or potential harms that mental illness poses. They describe different kinds of responses we must make, and why, in order to help people cope with their illness and promote resilience.

While social support is crucial for people with mental illness to be able to cope with their illness, and thus important for helping people to act in resilient ways, it is not by itself a sufficient response to mental illness. Resilience requires not only inner resources and social support, but also external resources and opportunities made available by institutions that can provide institutional support. After all, while vulnerabilities can be addressed in part through interpersonal means, they also require institutional aid and provision as well as structural justice. Justice approaches that focus on the responsibility that institutions have, both for meeting people's needs in a human rights context and for ensuring structural justice by addressing social determinants of mental health, are also necessary. I develop these approaches in chapters 5 and 6.

Chapter 5

Resources for Meeting People's Needs

Introduction

In Ken Steele's story, we see vividly how someone with severe mental health challenges is easily subjected to having their life structured around many different systems. Much of Steele's book describes his experiences with the mental health system, which had many components. These included the medical and psychiatric hospitals he stayed in (including both publicly funded state psychiatric hospitals and privately funded psychiatric hospitals), sometimes for months at a time; the residence facilities that provided halfway houses for him to live in; the rehabilitation programs that helped him find work and that helped structure his days; and the networks of mental health professionals (including psychiatrists and therapists) that he saw both as an inpatient and as an outpatient. In addition, when he was homeless, he had experiences in systems that support homeless and impoverished people, which overlapped with the mental health system in some areas. While Steele was never incarcerated, as a person with severe mental illness who was institutionalized and homeless for long periods of time, he could have easily also been subjected to the criminal justice system and its associated rehabilitative systems. As Steele's story illustrates, many people with severe mental illness interact with a variety of different systems designed to help them.

While Elyn Saks largely locates responsibility for her mental health within herself and in friends and mental health professionals working with her, as discussed in chapter 5, Steele locates responsibility at least partly within systems. In contrast to Saks's story, which focuses mostly on her interactions with other individuals, Steele's story focuses on interventions provided by institutions and systems that are designed to help people in need. Steele did not have the support of family and friends the way Saks did; he did not have a network of people he could rely on and so had to rely on the systems available to take care of the needy.

Steele's family abandoned him, and he was unable to make friends with people who were in a position to help him. After Steele started showing symptoms, his family wanted nothing to do with him. He describes being "divorced" by his parents who refused to see him or be there for him when he was ill.[1] While he occasionally made friends with other mental patients and homeless people, he never had the opportunity to make friends with people who lived more stable lives and could help provide more of a support system for him. His friends did provide him with some support, including at times emotional support, roommate situations, and job opportunities, but they were more limited in what they could do for him compared to Saks's friends, largely because they were situated very differently. While Saks's friends lived more stable, middle-class lives, and could draw on their resources to help her, Steele's friends were in significant need themselves and had far fewer resources to offer.

Thus, Steele mostly had to rely on institutions and systems to provide the resources he needed. For more than three decades, he cycled in and out of hospitals, long-term psychiatric institutions, residence care facilities, rehabilitation programs, and homelessness. He became a client of the mental health system, the disability system, and the systems addressing homelessness and poverty. He developed what he identified as a dependency on these systems, as he could not take care of himself on his own and he was unable to live independently for significant lengths of time.

Sometimes the interventions to which he was subjected were voluntary, but often they were not. Occasionally, he sought out help on his own, such as going to a hospital emergency room of his own accord or going to a shelter, but often he received help after being forced into it, such as when police officers brought him to a psychiatric hospital and hospitalized him. People who were part of institutions designed to help sometimes reached out to him to offer help, such as medical doctors and social workers who reached out to the homeless to offer mental health services, including the psychiatrist who wrote the foreword to his book, Stephen Mark Goldfinger. Sometimes Steele chose to take people up on their offer, and sometimes he didn't. Sometimes he wasn't given a choice.

People who lack social support networks and who do not have individuals in their lives who can offer the resources they need often have to rely on systems and institutions to provide those resources. Even people who do have support networks, however, often need to rely on systems in addition to relying on friends, family, and other individuals in their support networks. While Saks's story focuses mostly on her interactions with other individuals, she too had to rely on the mental health system for treatment, both during the times when she was hospitalized and during all the time she was under the care of a psychiatrist/psychoanalyst. The mental health system was essential for her to receive the treatment that she needed.

Many institutions are designed with the express purpose of helping people in certain kinds of need. Hospitals help sick people; psychiatric hospitals and other psychiatric institutions help mentally ill patients. Homeless shelters help the homeless; food banks help those who cannot feed themselves. Rehabilitation programs help people with mental illness get jobs and structure their days through day programs. The mental health system provides outreach and treatment to mentally ill people, including indigent people who do not have insurance or their own ways of getting mental health support. Disability services provide assistance to those who qualify as disabled. Even the criminal justice system provides assistance, including treatment and rehabilitation services in jails and prisons and through other criminal justice system channels such as drug courts.

Institutions meet people's needs by providing them with the resources and opportunities necessary for people to have autonomous agency and epistemic agency (especially meaning-making capacity). For people with mental illness, this primarily involves giving them access to mental health resources including education, outreach, and treatment. But, secondarily, it also involves giving them access to resources to meet other needs, including food, shelter, healthcare, and jobs. People who do not get their basic needs fulfilled not only experience constraints on their agency, autonomy, and meaning-making capacity, but they also experience poorer mental health due to the stressful conditions in which living without basic goods results. Meeting mental health needs thus requires meeting all of people's basic needs.

Meeting people's basic needs enables resilience in several ways. First, it provides people with tools they can use in trying to change their situation. The more resources a person can draw upon, the more options they have, which gives them more possibilities in trying to change their circumstances. Second, it provides people with tools they can use in trying to endure situations that are outside of their control. It is easier to endure difficult situations when a person only has one difficulty to focus on and get through; if their basic needs are met, then *that* aspect of their situation at least is not difficult.

Third, meeting people's basic needs gives people external resources to draw upon and rely upon in developing and channeling inner resources like skills, virtues, and attitudes. When a person already has their basic needs met, they don't have to spend precious time and energy worrying about how they will survive and scavenging for the resources they need. Instead, they can use their time and energy more productively, such as to focus on their loved ones, develop their talents and skills, and interact positively with others. This enables them more easily to develop the inner resources they need for being resilient.

As I have mentioned earlier, responsibility for mental health is often viewed in an individualistic lens, especially when the focus for addressing mental health is on individual resilience. In chapter 4, I showed how Elyn Saks viewed responsibility for her mental health in this way and then pointed out how the interactions of other individuals was also a necessary component to rebuilding her mental health in response to mental illness. Addressing mental illness and meeting mental health needs is thus partly individual and partly interpersonal. It is also, however, partly institutional, in several ways. I discuss the ways institutions enable or disable justice in chapter 6; here, I discuss the way they fulfill people's human rights by meeting their basic needs. Examining the nature of responsibility in a needs framework helps us to better understand the kinds of institutional responsibilities individuals have to address mental illness.

One of the ways responsibility for addressing mental health is institutional is that institutions specifically have the means—and duty—to provide the resources needed to address mental health. This chapter shows how addressing mental health needs is a human rights issue requiring institutional response. I argue that people have a right to mental health that can only be fulfilled through institutional responsibilities of providing appropriate and adequate resources that meet their mental health and other basic needs.

A Human Rights Approach to Mental Health

We see through Steele's experience that responsibility for addressing mental health needs is in part *institutional*. Institutions are required to meet people's mental health needs because they have more power and capacity to do so compared to individuals. Organized agencies working within systems can provide resources and opportunities for those in need to help get their needs met. Institutions that work with people who have mental illness have responsibilities to be both resourceful and just, so they can be effective in meeting people's mental health needs.

One way to understand institutional responsibility for meeting people's mental health needs is in terms of meeting people's human rights. While fulfilling human rights sometimes involves interpersonal action and forbearance, in what is called an interactional approach to human rights, it also often involves institutional action and forbearance, as in an institutional approach to human rights. For many if not all human rights, an interactional response is vastly insufficient, because individuals do not have enough power over other individuals' lives to be able to meet their human rights; an institutional response is usually required. Meeting the right to mental health and other basic rights requires an institutional approach.

A rights approach conceptualizes rights as grounded in basic needs. Alan Gewirth views basic needs as the elemental needs a person has to meet the requirements of what he calls purposive agency (or what I have been calling autonomous agency), which are freedom and well-being.[2] Every individual needs freedom and well-being in order to have and exercise purposive/autonomous agency. From a normative point of view, this personal need must be universalized for all human beings. Gewirth argues, "Every agent, on pain of self-contradiction, must also accept the generalization that all prospective purposive agents have the generic rights [to freedom and well-being]."[3] Like Miller, Gewirth regards Kantian universalizability as a key feature of a normative framework that grounds rights and responsibilities.

This universalizability of the needs for purposive agency leads to what Gewirth calls the Principle of Generic Consistency (PGC). The PGC sets a normative prescription based on needs for agency. This prescription states, "Act in accord with the generic rights of your recipients as well as of yourself."[4] The PGC requires that we meet people's rights to the goods needed for freedom and well-being, just as they must meet our rights to these goods, in order to enable people to maintain and exercise their agency, just as they enable us to do the same.

Gewirth identifies three kinds of goods required for agency: basic, nonsubtractive, and additive goods.[5] Basic goods are the goods that serve as preconditions for action, including "life, physical integrity, and mental equilibrium."[6] When these are threatened, people cannot exercise basic (minimal) agency. Nonsubtractive goods are abilities and conditions that a person needs to *maintain* their ability to pursue their self-chosen purposes, in other words to be able to act to achieve their self-chosen ends or goals. Rights to nonsubtractive goods are infringed upon when a person is prevented from being able to make future plans, set future goals, and take steps needed to achieve those goals, such as through lying, cheating, or resource deprivation.[7]

Additive goods are abilities and conditions that are necessary to *increase* a person's ability to pursue their self-chosen purposes. Goods such as self-esteem, education, and social identities are additive goods that can be threatened with affronts to self-esteem, restrictions on education, and discrimination.[8] While ample additive goods can enhance agency, some threshold of additive goods must be met in order for people to have minimal autonomous agency. The right to additive goods for the sake of improving agency can be seen as a spectrum right, in which people have a greater right to a minimal set of these goods that enable minimal autonomous agency, and a lesser right (but still some moral priority) to a more robust set of these goods that enable enhanced agency.

In recognizing mental equilibrium as one of the basic goods that are preconditions for action, Gewirth acknowledges the centrality of mental health to exercising basic human capacities. Mental health is also a nonsubtractive and additive good that is necessary for people to be able to determine values and goals and to pursue their self-chosen ends, enabling them both to maintain and to improve these capacities. When mental health is lacking, a person can lose the abilities to envision themselves in the future, conceptualize future goals, and discern what steps they must take to try to attain goals. Threats to mental health, such as mental illness, constrain a person's autonomous agency.

Mental health can be seen as a spectrum right just like additive goods. Mental health is a basic good insofar as people need to meet a threshold level of basic mental health in order to have minimal autonomous agency. For example, people need to be connected to reality in the right sort of way and have their emotions regulated sufficiently so that they can function in various life domains. Higher standards of mental health are often necessary for enhanced agency. The moral priority would be to meet people's basic mental health needs, but some moral weight should also be given to mental health needs required for increased agency.

The right to mental health is in fact recognized by the United Nations. In article 12 in part 3 of the International Covenant on Economic,

Social and Cultural Rights (1966), mental health is briefly mentioned: "The States Parties to the present Covenant recognize the right of everyone to the enjoyment of the highest attainable standard of physical and mental health."[9] What mental health consists in in this document is left open-ended. The goal of enjoying mental and physical health involves achieving "the highest attainable standard," meaning the greatest health possible given unavoidable constraints. These constraints likely include personal limitations given one's physiology and psychology and possibly social limitations set by the reality of finite resources. To the extent that one's biological and psychological makeup allows it, and to the extent that institutions have resources and support to offer to people in need, institutions are obligated to make strides in increasing people's mental and physical health.

It is remarkable that in 1966, mental health was treated with parity in comparison to physical health by the United Nations. Among the steps outlined in the Covenant involved in realizing the right to "the enjoyment of the highest attainable standard of physical and mental health" is this step: "The creation of conditions which would assure to all medical service and medical attention in the event of sickness."[10] Given that this step is included in the context of trying to achieve maximal mental and physical health, we can presume that mental health services and mental health attention partly comprise what constitutes medical services and medical attention. The United Nations thus affirms that people have a human right to receive mental health services that will increase their mental health to the extent possible given the reality of unavoidable constraints.

The significance of having a human right to mental health is that it enables people to make rights claims to attain resources and support that increase their mental health. Rights can be understood as entitlements; a human right grants people an entitlement to get their human right met. When something is the object of a human right, people are entitled to make claims upon individuals, nations, and institutions to secure access to that object.[11]

James Griffin argues that a right to health cannot *literally* be a right to health, because no one can guarantee someone's health; it is not within anyone's control. A right to health is a right to the provisions needed to gain or maintain health, some of which involve access to health care but also which involve things such as education, infrastructure, employment, and various types of support. A right to mental health is a welfare right in which one has the right to the provisions needed to gain or maintain mental health, including access to mental healthcare treatment, as well as education, employment, other types of meaningful activity, income, emotional support, and other types of resources and support. Since social harms, inadequate needs fulfillment, social marginalization, and oppression can all cause stress that leads to mental health problems, a right to mental health also entails that agents and institutions do not subject people to various kinds of injustices. I discuss this more in chapter 6.

A right to mental health is tightly connected with other rights that are founded on people's basic needs. Lacking other basic needs such as food, housing, healthcare, or employment can negatively impact mental health by causing stress and difficulty that can lead to depression, anxiety, mood swings, thought disorder, inattention, impulsive behavior, and other mental disorder symptoms. Meeting people's human right to mental health thus requires meeting people's human rights to other basic needs. Realizing the human right to mental health, therefore, requires providing the resources and opportunities necessary for realizing human rights to *all* basic needs.

Institutional Duties to Fulfill Human Rights

A human rights approach to mental health provides a justice framework for understanding the kinds of responsibilities that individuals and (more appropriately) institutions have for addressing mental health. In chapter 2, I described how mental illness makes people especially vulnerable, susceptible to both ontological and situational harms that exacerbate and compound each other. A human rights framework provides a way for understanding the kind of response that is needed for institutions to engage in to protect people from such vulnerabilities. A human rights approach generates strong obligations, including strong positive obligations, to realize human rights as a way of responding to the vulnerability and needs that human rights serve to protect.[12] Institutions bear the greatest responsibility in meeting people's human right to mental health because they have significant power and capacity to structure people's lives. Let us look at this more closely.

The right to mental health can be understood as involving multiple duties and different kinds of actions. Henry Shue argues that basic rights, which for him are security and subsistence rights, have three correlative duties: to avoid harming people (such as through deprivation, in the case of subsistence rights), to protect people from harm (or to protect people from deprivation), and to aid vulnerable people (or to assist those who are deprived).[13] All three of these kinds of duties are entailed by any basic right. Other duties, such as the duty to compensate for harms that have already been committed or harms that are unavoidable, may also be relevant.

In the context of mental health, these correlative duties can be understood as follows. First, the right to mental health entails the duty to avoid causing harm to people's mental health, for example by not subjecting them to extraordinarily stressful, unjust, or otherwise harmful conditions that can negatively impact their mental health. Second, the right to mental health entails the duty to protect people from being subject to these kinds of conditions and so to help prevent people from having their mental health worsened by their situation. Third, the right to mental health entails the duty to aid people who have poor mental health by providing them with the resources and opportunities that they need to address mental illness. This includes mental health outreach, education, and treatment; but also jobs, education, and day programs; as well as spiritual, existential, ecological, and other resources. Aiding people in these ways involves improving mental health; increasing functioning and enhancing basic human capacities like agency, autonomy, and meaning-making; and promoting resilience. Fourth, the right to mental health entails the duty to compensate people for harms to their mental health, such as stressful or unjust situations that create or worsen mental health difficulties, in ways that help ameliorate this harm.

All of these duties involve both positive and negative actions, or both actions and forbearance. The duty to avoid causing harm involves both refraining from inflicting harm on people, such as by refraining from coercing them into treatment, and finding ways to interact with people that do not inflict harm, such as providing ways for individuals to understand their treatment, make choices about their treatment, and give meaningful consent. The duty to protect people from being subject to harm involves both not allowing people or institutions to act in harmful ways, such as rules that prohibit the use of restraints; and actively stopping people or institutions from inflicting harm through interventions, such as intervening and redirecting in situations where a person may be subjected to violence. The duty to aid people with mental illness involves both providing goods and resources that can help improve their mental health—including the aforementioned mental health education, outreach, and treatment—and not interfering with their access to these goods and services. The duty to compensate for harm that is already committed or that is unavoidable involves both positive actions, such as giving money to people who have experienced abuse or trauma; and forbearance, such as letting people with mental illness go through the grievance process in a hospital that has caused them harm. Carrying out any of the duties correlated with the right to mental health requires both positive and negative actions to be taken.

Notice that many of these positive and negative actions not only protect people from vulnerability, but—when done well—also increase autonomous agency and epistemic agency. Avoiding causing harm, protecting people from harm, aiding, and compensating for harm can and ought all to be performed in ways that promote autonomous agency and epistemic agency by supporting the advancement of vulnerable individuals' own ends and increasing their understanding and meaning-making capacity. In these ways, such actions can avoid creating the pathogenic vulnerabilities that interventions sometimes cause.

While a human rights approach must involve both negative and positive obligations, Onora O'Neill challenges the concept of duties of assistance. She argues that such duties entail primarily positive actions that can be undertaken sometimes, in some circumstances, but not always, in all circumstances, thus making them constitute what Kant would call imperfect duties.[14] Furthermore, she argues that rights only have meaning if they specify the duty-bearer who is obligated to fulfill the right. Perfect duties, which tend to involve acts of forbearance or noninterference, are universal in scope, implicitly applying to everyone at all times, thus inherently specifying their duty-bearers. Imperfect duties, which tend to involve positive action, however, apply only to specific duty-bearers, not all duty-bearers, and so they must specify the relevant duty-bearers in order to be meaningful.

It is not enough to say that "some people" somewhere must carry out these actions, according to O'Neill; the specific people who have this duty must be identifiable so that the duty is assignable. But for a right like the right to mental health, or any of the welfare rights associated with meeting people's basic needs, it is not necessarily obvious who has the responsibility to carry out the associated duties of aid. "Some" people and institutions do, but which ones are not specified by the duty.

O'Neill's solution to this problem is to propose that for whatever imperfect duties are entailed by human rights, specific institutions must be designed with the express purpose of carrying out these duties and meeting the needs of people who can claim the relevant rights. In the context of mental illness, this means creating institutions that have as at least one of their express purposes to provide the aid needed to maintain or improve people's mental health. This requirement includes creating institutions to provide the mental health education, outreach, and treatment that are especially relevant to the duty of assisting the mentally ill. It also includes creating institutions to provide the jobs, education, housing, and other resources, activities, and opportunities necessary for people with mental illness to increase their basic human capacities such as agency, autonomy, and meaning-making.

I think O'Neill's proposal is a good solution in search of a problem. Because duties involve both positive and negative actions, it is too simplistic to identify the duty of aid as an imperfect duty. The duty of aid requires multiple kinds of actions, some of which involve negative actions of not interfering with people's secure access to the goods required for mental health, and some of which involve positive actions of providing certain goods and services that maintain or improve mental health. Such negative actions can be performed by everyone all the time, while such positive actions can only be performed by certain people or institutions some of the time. The duty to aid involves both kinds of actions and thus is not *merely* an imperfect duty as O'Neill conceptualizes it.

Furthermore, the positive actions involved with the duty to aid can be understood as actions that anyone situated in a certain way in relation to people's mental health needs is obligated to perform, making it a universal prescription that is contextualized. For example, anyone interacting with a person with mental illness who is in crisis has a duty to help the person access mental health resources, such as by connecting them with a therapist or psychiatrist. And everyone who is part of a social and political community that distributes resources to its citizens has a duty to advocate for mental health resources for the most vulnerable and needy. While people are not in a situation of responding to people in mental health crises or advocating for distribution of mental health resources all the time, they have the duty to respond at any time that they *are* in these situations.

Along these lines, Gewirth argues that the duties corresponding to basic human rights such as the right to mental health are universal in the sense that anyone who is situated in the right position must carry them out. He says, "The universality of a right, so far as concerns the duty it imposes, is not primarily a matter of everyone's actually fulfilling the duty, let alone doing so at all times. Nor is it even a matter of everyone's always being able to fulfill the duty. It is rather a matter of everyone's always having the duty to act accordingly when the circumstances arise which require such action and when he then has the ability to do so, this ability including consideration of costs to himself."[15] In other words, anyone who is in the right context is obligated to carry out the relevant action that is required given that context, making the duty universal.

O'Neill conceptualizes the duty of assistance wrongly, and she mistakenly does not recognize that even positive actions involved with the duty of assistance can be universal given their context, making the problem of claimability that she identifies not a genuine problem that needs fixing. Nevertheless, her proposed solution is an important consideration for understanding how such a duty can best be met. Institutions *should* be designed in such a way as to carry out the duties associated with the right to mental health in order to provide a specific way for this right to be fulfilled because they are the most appropriate agents who can do so.

In many contexts, the *best* agents to carry out duties correlated with the right to mental health are institutions, which can be understood as collective agents or "organized agencies"[16] (such as government agencies and nongovernmental organizations), and the social structures (such as the way work or welfare is structured in a given society) and systems (such as the mental health system, the criminal justice system, and the system to aid homeless people) in which institutions operate. This is because the collective agents or organized agencies involved with setting up and maintaining social structures and systems have considerably more power and organizational structure than individuals.

Institutions are able to collect and process information and compute consequences of actions more easily than individuals, so they can make better decisions. They have more resources to organize themselves effectively to carry out actions. They have greater capacity, power, and resources to effect change, so they can implement actions that individuals by themselves cannot do. In addition, they can distribute the costs involved with taking action so they can bear the burden of the cost more easily. In short, they can organize themselves and take action in ways that individuals cannot do alone.[17]

In the human rights literature, institutions are often identified as the primary bearers of responsibility for meeting human rights because they have the greatest capacity to do so. In addition to having capacity

Resources for Meeting People's Needs   141

to perform positive obligations, institutions have power over individuals and must be organized in such a way as to protect people from harm and avoid inflicting harm themselves. The ways that institutions condition individual action by making some options available and others not, and by providing the background context for how actions are understood and what meaning they are given, makes institutions especially powerful in individuals' lives, and so they have the responsibility to direct that power in protective and supportive ways.

For example, consider some of the ways that institutions condition the lives of those with mental illness. Institutions such as mental health treatment centers, including hospitals and outpatient clinics, shape the quality of treatment people can receive. If they are resourceful, they can help promote people's agency, autonomy, and meaning-making capacity in the course of treatment; if they are impoverished or unjust, they can perpetuate violence, abuse, neglect, exploitation, coercion, marginalization, oppression, and domination. Social structures such as the way work, welfare, and education are structured shape what opportunities are available to a person with mental illness. They can be resourceful in providing jobs that people with psychiatric disabilities can perform, providing access to appropriate levels of education, and connecting disabled people with income and health insurance. Or they can be impoverished in providing disabled people with few opportunities and resources they can access and even creating obstacles for people with mental illness to find jobs, access education, and pursue social resources.

Institutions that are designed for specific purposes have greater obligation and more specific responsibilities for fulfilling the duties associated with that purpose, while other institutions have more diffused responsibilities of providing ways for individuals to interface with the institution justly and well. For example, institutions that are designed to aid people with mental health problems and related vulnerabilities, such as hospitals and work skills centers, have a stronger obligation and a wider array of responsibilities related to their interactions with such vulnerable people. Institutions that have other purposes, on the other hand, such as utility or delivery companies, have a narrower range of responsibilities and more diffused responsibility, such as the responsibilities associated with helping a person in a mental health crisis when such a person is encountered.

Mental health systems, the disability system, systems addressing homelessness, and the criminal justice system also shape what options for action people with mental illness have. When these systems are resourceful, individuals are able to find and access the resources and opportunities they need to be able to be successful; when these systems are impoverished or unjust, people encounter obstacles to finding and accessing resources and opportunities, and they may be subject to harms such as stigma, prejudice, discrimination, abuse, violence, neglect, exploitation, coercion, marginalization, domination, and oppression. How institutions, structures, and systems are organized, what resources they have available, and what opportunities they can create all impact greatly the living conditions of those with mental illness.

Depending on how they are structured, institutions have significant capacity and power to inflict harm, protect from harm, compensate for harm, or provide aid. Individuals are thus vulnerable to the power institutions have over their lives, as I discussed with respect to social-structural vulnerability in chapter 2. They are at risk of being harmed by institutions, even institutions that are designed to protect them, when the institutions create pathogenic vulnerabilities. Individuals are also dependent on institutions to provide the resources and opportunities they need to be able to exercise agency, autonomy, and meaning-making capacity. Individuals cannot exercise these human capacities without the influence of institutions because institutions, structures, and systems always serve as the backdrop for, and thus always condition and shape, human action and experience. Individual experience and action are *always* influenced by institutions, structures, and systems. Institutions thus have significant power to aid, protect, support, or harm individuals.

While some of the harms that institutions, structures, and systems are capable of inflicting are additive, contributing one more harm to a person's overall burden, many harms are multiplicative, magnifying the harms a person already experiences so they are much worse than they were prior to institutional intervention.[18] As noted in chapter 2, the vulnerabilities people with mental illness experience are compounding, meaning they inherently lead to other vulnerabilities because of the way harms are linked structurally and systemically. Some of these compounding harms add additional burden, such as discrimination that closes off certain options, while others magnify harms already experienced, such as lack of access and opportunity that leads to homelessness that then makes it difficult for a person to get a job or eat. With their significant power over individuals' lives, institutions have the ability to inflict many harms that are not only additive but also multiplicative.

The power of institutions to condition and shape individuals' lives leads to several kinds of institutional responsibilities. Institutions that inflict harm on individuals, or that allow harm to occur without stopping it, have a responsibility to reform themselves so they do not cause or allow harm. Unjust institutions must be reformed so they are more just; institutions that allow violence, abuse, neglect, stigma, or prejudice must be changed so these no longer occur. Institutions have a responsibility to take action to protect individuals from harm, such as by creating rules and policies that safeguard individuals and providing resources and opportunities that allow individuals to evade potential harm. They also have a responsibility to compensate for harm that has already been committed or that is unavoidable.

In addition, institutions have a responsibility to aid and support individuals by providing as many resources and opportunities as possible so that individuals may develop and exercise their agency, autonomy, and meaning-making capacity. This means providing jobs; education access; safe and stable housing; mental health education, outreach, and treatment; access to medical treatment; and meaningful activities that help a person structure their day in ways that support individuals' fundamental human capacities. Institutions must promote agency, autonomy, and meaning-making in the ways that they are designed so they can support individuals in maintaining or improving these important human capacities.

Fulfilling people's human right to mental health also requires offering the resources that people need in order to be resilient in the face of mental health and life challenges. In addition to material and social resources, the institutional duty to provide resources to vulnerable people also involves supplying other kinds of resources, like spiritual, existential, and ecological resources that a person can draw upon in responding to adversity. To help individuals be resilient, institutions must provide an array of resources that both meet people's basic needs and enable resilience.

In the context of mental illness, all institutions that condition the lives of people with mental illness—including those related to the mental health system, but also all the other systems mentioned here—have these institutional responsibilities. In fact, all institutions where individuals may interact with people who have mental illness—which probably includes any institution one can think of—have institutional responsibilities to shape interaction so that it is protective, supportive, respectful, noncoercive, autonomy-promoting, epistemic agency–promoting, and just. In this way, institutions can help fulfill people's human right to mental health.[19]

The Responsive State

Fulfilling people's human rights by meeting their basic needs, including their mental health needs, is one of the responsibilities of what Martha Albertson Fineman calls "the responsive state."[20] The role of the responsive state is to protect people from vulnerability, and it does this in part by intentionally designing institutions to support people and protect them from vulnerability. This is the state (government) that forms in response primarily to our inherent ontological vulnerabilities, according to Fineman, but also to our situational vulnerabilities. In the responsive state, institutions are designed to respond to people's vulnerabilities by protecting them from the harms to which they are at risk. A sufficiently responsive state is a robust state that prioritizes distributive and structural justice and is thus incompatible with libertarian ideals of a minimal state.

Because of the power of institutions to influence and shape our experience and action, we create institutions to help us deal with our vulnerability. In this way, we try to exert control over our risk of harm. Bryan Turner argues that we create social institutions—which include the organized agencies, social structures, and systems discussed earlier—in order to try to deal with our precarity, insecurity, and uncertainty.[21] Because our lives are marked by so much risk of harm and adversity, we try to create structures that help mitigate or prevent harm. In this way, we try to compensate for the fundamental lack of control we have over what happens to us by controlling the social conditions that are the background of our experience and action. Society is thus created in response to the potential harms that all humans face, in order to provide protection, support, and resources that allow individuals to withstand or avoid harms.

When we have social institutions that respect and enforce human rights; provide healthcare, education, and employment; provide assistance; allow us to litigate against wrongdoings; and pursue justice, we create social conditions that prevent or mitigate the harm that always threatens to overtake us. Through social institutions, we try to deal with our vulnerability by finding ways to protect ourselves from the precarity, insecurity, and uncertainty that pervades our lives. The responsive state arises from this need to protect ourselves and one another from vulnerability. In a vulnerability model, the universal ontological vulnerability of human beings grounds responsibilities of the state.

The responsive state is a way of reallocating responsibilities so they are not primarily the obligation of individuals in need and the individuals who interact with them, but rather the obligation of the society and government that are responsible for their citizens.[22] In this way, it makes individuals dependent and interdependent on their government and its associated institutions, rather than on other individuals. Thus, it is a way of organizing society so that individuals get their needs met and are protected from harm by institutions, structures, and systems that have the power and capacity to support and protect.

In creating institutions that are designed to carry out the responsibilities required for protecting people from harm, we fulfill our responsibility to each other to take care of each other. Our vulnerabilities create in us deep needs that we are unable to meet by ourselves. We need to rely on others with whom we share relationships of interdependence so that others can meet our needs. But we are unable to meet each other's needs simply through interpersonal interactions; some needs cannot be met by specific others, for a variety of reasons. What is needed are institutions that can meet people's needs through collective action and through the members of the institution carrying out roles related to the institution's responsibility for meeting people's needs. Some needs can be met only through the organized action of institutions. Taking care of each other by meeting people's needs requires us to design institutions that have this responsibility as their primary function and that are organized to be able to carry out the specific duties involved with this general responsibility effectively. Only in this way can we effectively take care of each other.

For people who are especially vulnerable due to how they are socially situated, it may be necessary to design institutions specifically to meet these special needs. In addition, existing institutions may need to direct their attention and action more carefully to meet the needs of those who are especially vulnerable. For people with mental illness, this means the responsive state is obligated to develop social institutions that mitigate the harms brought about by mental illness, both the ontological harms that are directly caused by mental illness—the harms to mind and body that threaten people's lives and agency—as well as the social harms that are the result of people's lived experience with mental illness. Enhancing the agency of people with mental illness and helping them to flourish requires us to work on increasing their functioning, both the mental and physical functioning that is threatened by mental illness symptoms and the social functioning related to how they are able to live in the world, interacting with others, while having mental illness.

Special institutions can be created for the express purpose of meeting the needs of this especially vulnerable population. For example, agencies that help people with mental illness find work in the community or mental health treatment centers that medically and psychologically treat mental illness exist for the primary purpose of aiding people with mental illness. In addition, existing institutions that respond to vulnerability more broadly can be directed to focus special attention and energy on the needs of those who are especially vulnerable. For example, health and human services agencies that help people with mental illness connect to mental health treatment and hospitals that respond to mental health crises through crisis management are designed to address the needs of people who have many different kinds of vulnerabilities, but they also give special attention and energy to the specific needs of mentally ill people.

In order for the responsive state to be effective at protecting people from vulnerability, institutions need to provide *adequate* resources, support, and opportunities. Providing substandard resources, support, and opportunities results in institutions not being able to meet people's needs and not being able to prevent or mitigate harm. Rather than protecting people from vulnerability, insufficient resources, support, and opportunities can actually exacerbate the vulnerability people already face or introduce new vulnerabilities caused by inadequate institutions, creating pathogenic vulnerabilities. When institutions are discriminatory, marginalizing, oppressive, coercive, exploitative, dominating, or otherwise unjust, this can exacerbate vulnerability or cause new vulnerabilities as well. The pathogenic vulnerabilities provided by insufficiently resourced or unjust institutions can create harm that is not offset by whatever help they are designed to give.

Impoverished or unjust institutions can exacerbate vulnerability or cause new vulnerabilities in many ways. For example, underfunded social agencies designed to help house people with severe mental illness may provide housing in dangerous areas, which is cheaper but which threatens the health and safety of people who are already vulnerable. Underfunded hospitals and crisis centers may not have the money to be able to intervene effectively in mental health crises, exacerbating the danger mentally ill people in crisis experience. Mental health staff in a psychiatric hospital who abuse patients create new vulnerabilities and harms, including trauma, in their patients. When employers make it hard for people with mental illness to access the healthcare treatment they need (such as through inflexible work hours), this exacerbates the difficulty already vulnerable people face in getting their healthcare needs met. Institutions must be resourceful and just in order to help meet people's needs adequately, in ways that are supportive and protective rather than incurring further harms.

What resourceful and just institutions can do, Fineman argues, is enable resilience, which she defines as addressing and confronting adversity.[23] She identifies five kinds of assets or resources that social institutions can provide to aid people in being able to be resilient. These include physical assets, such as housing, food, transportation, and consumer items; human resources, including human capital, education, training, knowledge, and experience; social networks, including not only family and close friends but also community membership and identity group membership; ecological resources, which encompass all of the natural environment, including clean air and water; and existential assets, which involve beliefs, aesthetics, religion, culture, art, and politics, and are the source of meaning and beauty.[24] In providing these resources, institutions help give individuals the tools to prevent and mitigate harm—both ontological harms and situational harms—and to maintain and improve their basic human capacities like agency, autonomy, and meaning-making. This list of resources is helpful to understand the range of resources that individuals need to be resilient.

Part of what institutions do in preventing and ameliorating harms and helping people to get their needs met is to assess and address systems of power, the privilege and disadvantages that people have based on how they are socially situated.[25] Systems of power and privilege create "webs of advantages and disadvantages"[26] that must be understood, untangled, and adjusted so that power and privilege are more evenly distributed. In a vulnerability approach, institutions and systems are brought "under scrutiny, redirecting our attention to their role in providing assets in ways that may unfairly privilege certain persons or groups, even if unintentionally."[27] In recognizing the role that institutions and systems play in perpetuating inequalities and injustices, we can address some of the situational vulnerabilities to which people are subject and avoid creating pathogenic vulnerabilities.

People who are especially vulnerable to situational vulnerabilities because of how they are positioned in society and to pathogenic vulnerabilities because of how they are positioned in relation to institutions and systems that have the power to harm them are in special need of responsive institutions set up within a responsive state. Because they are especially disadvantaged, in multiple compounding and interlocking ways, they stand to benefit the most from investigating the roles that institutions and systems play in allowing or perpetuating inequalities and injustices. Those who are especially vulnerable, such as people who have disabilities (including psychiatric disabilities) or people who have mental illness, require special attention and special interventions in order to receive the same amount of protection as everyone else in order to get their human rights met.[28]

Fineman notes that the state plays a central role in enabling institutions to offer these resources. She says, "Many of the institutions providing resources that give us resilience can only be brought into legal existence through state mechanisms."[29] For example, institutions and structures such as corporations, schools, workplaces, families, and churches are all legitimized by the state and are given status that confers benefits and protections by the law.[30] Fineman proposes that we reconceptualize the role of the state as one that empowers vulnerable subjects (who comprise all of its citizens, and especially those who face more and greater vulnerabilities) by creating responsive structures that can create an equitable distribution of assets and privilege.[31] This produces greater equality, encourages public participation, and helps shore up democracy.[32]

While institutions are designed to protect people from both universal and situational vulnerabilities and to meet people's universal human rights, they must also be designed to carry out their duties in particular, context-specific ways. Thus, while they fulfill universal needs, they must do so in variable ways that are appropriate to whatever specific contexts there are. People who are occurrently in need are subject to occurrent harm that must be addressed immediately, while people who are dispositionally in need are subject to risk of harm that can be addressed in a less immediate way. The particular situational vulnerabilities and pathogenic vulnerabilities to which people are subject must be addressed by looking at and reforming the specific institutions and systems involved. Ensuring that people get their needs met requires responding to their particular circumstances and individualizing response based on this. Thus, meeting people's universal basic needs and fulfilling their universal human rights—which some people can already meet within existing social circumstances, but which others can't—requires responses that are particular and context-specific.

Human rights are best met by institutions, which can be designed to meet people's needs effectively and justly by fulfilling their human rights without imposing additional pathogenic vulnerabilities, in ways that promote people's basic human capacities like agency and autonomy. It is the responsibility of the state to design institutions and systems that prevent and mitigate harm, protecting people from vulnerability. They do this by providing a range of resources that help people get their needs met and allow them to develop and exercise their basic human capacities, including agency, autonomy, and meaning-making capacity. In this way, they provide the resources and opportunities that people need to draw upon and mobilize in changing or adapting to their situation in order to be resilient.

With their organizational power, capacity, and reservoir of resources, institutions are the agents best positioned to carry out the correlative duties associated with the right to mental health. These include duties to provide mental health education, outreach, and treatment, as well as access to general medical treatment, in a way that increases agency and autonomy and avoids coercion, violence, and other harms. Other duties of aid include providing opportunities for jobs and education, providing access to disability services, and providing safe and stable housing, all in ways that increase people's agency and autonomy without belittling them, stigmatizing or discriminating against them, or otherwise harming them. Other resources institutions are obligated to provide in order to help individuals be resilient in the face of mental health and life challenges include spiritual, existential, and ecological resources. By providing these resources and enabling people to be more resilient, institutions help fulfill individuals' right to mental health.

In addition, institutions have duties to create safeguards, policies, and interventions that protect people with mental illness from coercion, violence, discrimination, and other harms. They have duties to compensate for harm that has already been committed or that is unavoidable. And, of course, they have duties to recognize when harms occur and be committed to avoiding inflicting harm, however unintentionally. I discuss these duties more in the context of structural justice in chapter 6.

States have obligations not only to protect people who already have mental illness through the activity of institutions that help govern individuals' lives, but also to protect people from developing mental illness by addressing some of the structural causes of mental illness. For example, in order to decrease people's risk of developing mental disorders, states need to provide adequate physical and mental healthcare, safe and stable housing, adequate minimum wages, various kinds of welfare safety nets, and other forms of social infrastructure. I discuss this more in chapter 6 when I discuss structural justice as a way to address the social determinants of mental health.

Empowering Agents to Get Their Human Rights Met

While institutions are the primary duty-bearers responsible for fulfilling people's human rights, individuals play a role, too. In chapter 4, I argued that *how* other people interact with a person with mental illness can deeply affect the person's mental state and enable them to be helped or harmed, depending on the quality of interaction. Similarly, how other people interact with an individual can determine the degree to which the individual gets their right to mental health met; other people can cause extremely stressful or unjust conditions that damage mental health, or they can be supportive, welcoming, and helpful. They can be indifferent, ignoring crisis situations, or they can be compassionate, trying to connect a person to resources and treatment.

However, it is not only other people interacting with those who have mental illness who have a responsibility to meet the mental health needs of people with mental illness. It is also the people with mental illness themselves. In the human rights literature, it has recently been recognized that the people who are most in need of getting their basic rights met still have agency, however compromised it may be due to not having their basic needs met, and consequently share a certain kind of responsibility for helping themselves.[33] While other agents, including institutions, have more capacity to help than the needy themselves, the needy still have agency and can take certain actions on their own behalf.

In other words, while they are in need, they do not need other agents to do *everything* for them to meet their human rights; there are certain actions they can—and *should*—take themselves. Earlier, we established that the ultimate end to making rights claims and getting one's human rights met is to maintain or increase purposive agency, in Gewirth's words, or autonomous agency, in my words. If this is so, then finding ways for the needy to exercise their agency in relation to their problems is essential.

In the context of mental health, this means that people with mental illness need to be actively involved with addressing their mental health challenges and not simply rely on other people, institutions, or systems to help them. This requires them to develop some independence in relation to their problems, in contrast to the dependence on others and on systems to meet their needs that sometimes occurs. As mentioned in chapter 2, Ken Steele lamented the fact that many people with severe mental illness become dependent on the mental health system (and other systems) and learn to rely on it, rather than themselves, to get their needs met. Part of developing the agency that is a fundamental human capacity and an ultimate end of all of our action requires that people learn some independence and develop some ways to take care of themselves.

People who are in need have special knowledge of their situation, which can make them more effective agents.[34] People with mental illness have firsthand knowledge about their experience with mental illness and treatment and about what is good for them: what they need and what approaches best help them.[35] More specifically, they have special knowledge of their symptoms, how they respond to particular treatments, how mental illness affects their functioning in various life domains, what kinds of accommodations they desire and have access to, and what psychological characteristics they need to employ to deal with their mental illness.[36] This special knowledge allows people with mental illness to understand their experience in a way that others may not be able to, recognizing what is morally salient about their situation and using this to develop frameworks of meaning that more accurately reflect their experience.

The special knowledge that individuals in need have of their experience and their situation is an important epistemic resource they can draw on and use in figuring out how to act. This helps them to exercise moral agency to change and control their situation. In addition, this special knowledge is a resource they can share with others who have the power and capacity to help them. When agents and institutions seek to understand the experience and perspective of people in need from their own point of view, people in need can share their special knowledge so that others can help them more effectively. In this way, they contribute to the work that is done on their behalf. When people with mental illness act as agents in working on getting their own right to mental health met, they play a role in effecting the change they would like to see.

In order for vulnerable individuals to be effective at sharing their special knowledge and voicing their needs, they need to be adequately listened to and responded to by the individuals and institutions that have power to help them. In other words, individuals' perspectives and concerns must be taken up appropriately by those who have the power to respond. Appropriate uptake is a matter of social justice, and deep listening and responsivity are crucial to uptake. I develop this more in chapter 6.

When people in need play an active role in getting their needs met, their goal is not *simply* to obtain the resources and opportunities required to fulfill their human rights. In the context of mental illness, their goal in meeting their right to mental health is not just to access treatment in order to address their mental illness. It also includes addressing the myriad harms and vulnerabilities that mental illness brings, including the need to get other basic needs met, as well as stigma, prejudice, coercion, abuse, violence, and various injustices. Their demands may include an end to social marginalization and exclusion[37] and a rectification of and compensation for injustice. They cannot simply wait and let institutions accomplish these goals for them; they must actively work toward these goals themselves and help institutions to help them by giving them the knowledge and understanding that institutions need to carry out their duties to meet people's mental health needs. In this way, vulnerable individuals can act as agents in working toward getting their own needs met by working with the institutions that are the primary duty-bearers for meeting those needs.

Conclusion

As we see in Steele's story, people with severe mental illness often interact with many systems and many institutions working within systems. The quality of the institutions matter; how resourceful and just an institution or system is affects how much benefit an individual gains from it. Institutions and systems can be helpful or harmful. Steele's experiences with coercion, restraints, horrific violence by fellow patients, and callous indifference by staff (all detailed in chapter 2) show that institutions can be harmful when they are not designed to protect patients from harm. Systems that are not autonomy-promoting can create dependence, which Steele says is common in people with severe mental illness who learn to rely on the mental health system without learning how to meet their own mental health needs themselves.

On the other hand, Steele benefited from some of the institutions he engaged with. He obtained jobs and housing from rehabilitation programs. The medication that ultimately made his voices cease, and helped him recover, was prescribed to him by a psychiatrist. As an outpatient, he saw therapists that helped him gain insight into his condition, which gave him more control over his situation. He was helped by many mental health workers who connected or provided him with treatment that helped him deal with his voices. Some aspects of the mental health system—and the related rehabilitative, disability, and homeless systems that overlapped with the mental health system—were very beneficial in Steele's life.

Though Steele may not have seen it this way, he, like all people, had a right to mental health, a right premised on the basic need for mental health in enabling him to exercise basic human capacities like agency, autonomy, and meaning-making. Other individuals did not have the power and capacity to fulfill his right to mental health adequately, but institutions and systems designed to address mental illness and its associated harms did. To some extent, institutions were able to give him some of the resources he needed to be able to live with his illness and be resilient in relation to it. On the other hand, many of the institutions he dealt with were too impoverished to give him *adequate* resources to be able to deal with his illness, which is why he struggled so severely for several decades. When they were impoverished or unjust, institutions not only failed to meet his right to mental health, but they actually caused him greater harm, worsening his mental health. When institutions were resourceful and just, however, they were effective in helping to get his mental health needs met.

A responsive state is a government that is set up to help protect people from the inherent ontological vulnerabilities we all face as well as the situational vulnerabilities that some people experience based on how they are socially situated. It creates institutions that protect people by meeting their various needs and providing them with the resources and opportunities that they need to mobilize in order to be resilient. The responsive state requires that we intentionally design institutions and systems with which people with mental illness interact to care for them properly by being respectful, noncoercive, autonomy-promoting, adequately resourced, and just.

In chapter 6, I look at another way that responsibility for addressing mental health is institutional: in the way that addressing mental health requires remedying structural injustices and ensuring social justice. Institutions do not just have the responsibility to provide adequate resources to meet people's human right to mental health (and other welfare rights predicated on basic needs). They also have the responsibility to be organized in a way that ensures justice. Making institutions more just also plays a pivotal role in addressing mental health and helping people with mental illness to be more resilient in the face of their illness and other life challenges.

Chapter 6

Resources for Social Justice

Introduction

Throughout his illness, Ken Steele was subject to many social injustices, some of which had a structural component, which exacerbated his mental illness. As a young adult recently moved to New York City, he was groomed for sexual exploitation. Without a job or a secure place to live, he was easily taken advantage of by people who gave him what he needed—income and a place to live—in exchange for working as a prostitute. He agreed to work as a prostitute only because he couldn't see that he had any other options to support himself. His family had disowned him, and at this point in his life he was unable to obtain or keep a regular paying job. So he was easily exploited by a private market system that takes advantage of people's needs to offer them certain kinds of work that they may be unable to refuse.[1] This experience dramatically worsened his mental health, making him extremely suicidal, and making the voices that he heard much more insistent.[2]

Later on, after several hospitalizations, he became homeless when he did not have a way to obtain gainful employment.[3] Homelessness is a social injustice that results from inefficiencies in the private housing market that rewards some people, those with adequate income and employment, and punishes others, those who lack this income and employment. We could have a system where all people are guaranteed safe and adequate housing, regardless of income, but we do not.[4] Instead, there are winners and losers of the system we have.

Once a person is homeless, it is very difficult for them to obtain a job, because they do not have an address to report, or in some cases (when they lack a cellphone)[5] a means to be contacted. Again, we could have a system that guarantees a job for all people, or at least provides a guaranteed income,[6] so that people would have the means to participate in systems like the private housing market, but, again, we do not. While unemployed (as Steele was when he was homeless), it was also difficult for Steele to receive outpatient mental healthcare, because, without a job, he lacked the health insurance that would pay for healthcare. In addition, while he was homeless, he was cut off from other systems that would have helped him support himself, such as the employment system under capitalism and the health insurance system that enables healthcare access.

During these periods, Steele suffered from social injustices in that he lacked power and received disproportionate and unjust burdens from structures that benefited and empowered others. Being subjected to social injustices worsened his mental health. Without a job to distract him and keep him tethered to reality, his voices intensified and his connection to reality thinned. Being homeless and downtrodden, his self-esteem plummeted, and he had little motivation to work to try to improve his condition. Without access to outpatient mental healthcare, he lacked the means to remedy his mental health without getting stuck in the inpatient mental health system. Instead, for decades, he cycled through homelessness and hospitalizations, often unable to access the housing and employment markets that would have enabled him to support himself.

At times, social structures did support him. In some places, he received rehabilitative services upon discharge from hospitals, and these helped connect him with a place to live (in halfway homes) and a job (such as working as a cook or an orderly).[7] During these times, his self-esteem increased, and he was proud of being able to support himself. When receiving rehabilitative services, he was also able to access mental healthcare, which alleviated his voices to some extent. By the time he was taking Risperdal (which was the only drug that ever eliminated the voices), he was living in his own apartment, through a housing subsidy for disabled people, and working. He was rightfully proud of being able to support himself, but he was only able to do so because of the presence of social institutions that provided him access to housing, employment, and healthcare. He would not have been able to access these on his own in the private markets. He relied on institutional help.

Institutions are not always just, even when they provide access to needed resources. Sometimes they can be the sites of coercion, abuse, or violence. Both Steele and Elyn Saks suffered from extensive coercion when they were institutionalized, including involuntary hospitalization, forcible injection of medication, and the use of body restraints.[8] As people with mental illness, and as mental patients receiving mental healthcare treatment, they were not trusted to be able to make decisions for themselves while they were institutionalized.

In addition, Steele experienced severe abuse and violence at times while institutionalized. He was the victim of rape, in a context where staff were aware of what patients were doing but did nothing to stop them.[9] He observed many fights, where staff not only condoned the violence but even seemed to egg it on,[10] and only protected himself from violence by developing an attitude and appearance of being someone one would not want to mess with. As a tall and large man, he was already an imposing figure, but he dealt with the violence all around him by trying to look and act intimidating so that others would not engage him in the violence. Institutions can allow significant injustice to occur when they are not organized in ways that empower the individuals whose lives they govern.

As we see from Steele's story, some people with mental illness experience many compounding situational vulnerabilities that exacerbate each other, contributing to further mental health problems. When Steele was young, unemployment and lack of stable housing led to sexual and economic exploitation, which led to worsened psychosis. Later, homelessness, unemployment, and lack of mental healthcare were all linked together, leading to such severe mental illness that Steele cycled between hospitalization and homelessness. Within the institutional setting, coercion, abuse, and violence were connected, each enabling the other by producing an environment where these were normalized. In these ways, Steele experienced linked social injustices caused at least in part by how institutions and systems were structured.

In order to be able to deal with his mental illness effectively, Steele needed help from institutions in at least two ways. He needed institutions and systems to be designed to enable him to have access to resources like housing, jobs, and healthcare, and he needed the institutions and systems with which he interacted to be organized in ways that were structurally just, with mechanisms that empowered him rather than dominating or oppressing him. When the systems around him were structurally just, this gave him more resources to draw upon in exercising his agency and autonomy, and in being resilient and dealing with his mental illness effectively. When they were unjust, they imposed constraints on his behavior and made achieving resilience much more difficult. Systems and institutions must be just in order for the vulnerable people whose lives they structure to have enough agency and autonomy to be resilient in the face of life challenges.

In this chapter, I examine what kind of responsibility institutions and individuals have to make institutions and systems more just, in order to address the situational vulnerabilities that result from unjust structures and to provide people with mental illness the resources they need to be resilient. Addressing situational vulnerabilities requires taking a social justice approach that examines the power relationships between differently situated groups of people. While social justice partly involves distributive justice, or ensuring adequate access to needed resources and opportunities, it also partly involves structural justice. Structural justice looks at how social structures position different groups of people to see if there are structural inequalities and power differentials inherent to their positioning that lead to forms of domination or oppression; when there are, institutions and systems need to be transformed to minimize inequalities of power and to be more just.

One aspect of social justice that involves transforming power relationships so they are more just is justice in uptake, where institutions are designed to have mechanisms to listen to the needs of the people whose lives they structure and make adjustments and improvements based on this feedback. Justice in uptake requires that institutions and systems position individuals in ways that grant them epistemic power, where they will be listened to and taken seriously, as well as moral power, in provoking action on the part of institutions in accordance with individuals' claims and testimony. In listening and being appropriately responsive, institutions can empower the individuals whose lives they govern, enabling them to have greater agency and autonomy. This allows individuals to be more resilient in the face of life challenges, and it transforms the power relationships between institutions and the individuals whose lives they structure to be more just.

To examine the way that addressing situational vulnerabilities and meeting mental health needs in part requires a social justice approach, we need first to understand what some of the contributing factors to poor mental health are. Biological factors certainly play a role, at least for some people. But social factors do as well. Sometimes social factors are the predominant causal factors; often, biological factors manifest only when they are triggered by the presence of social factors. To better understand the role of social factors, let us look at social determinants of mental health.

Social Determinants of Mental Health

Social determinants of mental health are the social conditions that structure the lives of people in ways that contribute to mental health problems. Ruth S. Shim and Michael T. Compton define the social determinants of health as "the conditions into which people are born, live, and age that are shaped by policy decisions and distribution of opportunity within societies."[11] It is not only distribution of opportunity, of course, but also distribution of resources that matters. What resources and opportunities people have access to shapes what kinds of options they have for action and what kinds of choices they can make, thus structuring what kinds of lives they can live.

Some of the social determinants of mental health include economic factors, living conditions, life experiences, social position, and environmental factors.[12] Economic factors include income inequality, poverty, under- and unemployment, job insecurity, and low levels of education. Living conditions that are factors include low quality housing, housing instability, lack of safety, neighborhood deprivation, food insecurity, insufficient nutrition, and inadequate access to healthcare. Life experiences that are factors include childhood neglect or abuse, other adversity experienced in youth, and various forms of trauma. Social position factors include discrimination, social exclusion, and racism. Environmental factors include adverse aspects of the built environment as well as fallout from climate change, pollution, and other environmental problems. All of these factors contribute to people developing both physical and mental health problems.

These social factors contribute to poor mental health by causing chronic stress, which negatively impacts areas of the brain that affect mental functioning.[13] Chronic stress leads to both physical and mental health problems, including high blood pressure, obesity, and heart problems, as well as mental disorder symptoms like despair, anxiety, feelings of worthlessness or defeat, and suicidal ideation, leading to mental disorders such as depression and anxiety disorders. Stress also exacerbates existing mental health problems, worsening conditions such as psychosis and mood disorders. Social factors such as those previously listed create extremely stressful and unjust conditions that pose challenges to mental health.

In addition to causing stress, these social factors structure how people are able to live their lives, reducing what options for action are available to them, thus restricting their agency.[14] Poor living conditions, socioeconomic conditions, environmental conditions, and social conditions provide fewer resources to people and less opportunity. People get caught in lives that feel stuck, because they feel like they have few or no options. These constraints on their agency cause significant distress, which also negatively impacts mental health.

Negative social factors increase mental health problems and decrease quality of life. The social outcomes of mental illness arise as a consequence of failed policy and social actions that hurt people with mental illness; they are not inevitable outcomes of mental illness. For example, Shim and Compton argue that in schizophrenia, joblessness and homelessness are not inevitable outcomes of the disease but rather occur as a result of social norms and public policies that are stigmatizing and discriminatory.[15] People with schizophrenia are often seen as unfit to work and are thus treated as such, leading to exclusion from the workforce, impacting housing security, food security, and other living conditions. If people with schizophrenia were viewed as having something valuable to contribute to society, and jobs were designed in ways that allowed them to use the abilities they have, they could be included in the workforce, leading to better living conditions.

Social determinants of mental health form the basis of many basic needs. Some of these basic needs include the requirements for physical survival, such as food (which satisfies a need for nutrition), water, clothing, safe and stable housing (which satisfies a need for shelter), and a source of income to be able to purchase needed goods. These requirements for physical survival or subsistence also enable agency. Some of these basic needs include requirements for security, such as physical safety, positive environmental conditions (such as clean air and water), and supportive built environments. Other basic needs include requirements for autonomous agency, such as adequate employment, a moderate level of education, and access to healthcare, including mental healthcare. Being in just and moral power relations relative to others—where one is not subject to social injustices like stigma, prejudice, discrimination, racism, sexism, and heterosexism—is also important.

Addressing social determinants of mental health requires two kinds of responses. Taking a human rights approach, as we did in chapter 5, is a form of distributive justice. Distributive justice occurs when resources are distributed among people in a fair way, such as by ensuring that all people have at least a certain threshold of necessary goods. In a distributive justice approach, people must get their basic needs met, and institutions

Resources for Social Justice 161

must be designed to fulfill this function. Having one's basic needs fulfilled goes a long way toward protecting people from mental health problems. Institutions have duties of aid to provide the resources needed to fulfill people's basic needs, and individuals have duties to protect the vulnerable that require them to contribute to the effort of fulfilling people's basic needs in whatever way they can.

Another response, which we are focusing on in this chapter, involves structural justice. To a large extent, the social determinants of mental health are a matter of structural injustice, resulting from injustices in the ways that institutions and systems work. While distributive justice looks simply at outcomes, structural justice looks at the processes involved that led to those outcomes, focusing particularly on structural processes. In the structural justice approach, a lack of basic needs being met is not simply a matter of bad luck or biological determinism, but instead is the result of unjust practices.

To achieve structural justice, the behavior of individuals and the practices of institutions must be changed so they are more just. In the context of mental health, this means that institutions, systems, and structures must be reformed to be more just so that they do not produce the injustices that currently comprise many of the social determinants of mental health. Institutions, systems, and individuals have duties of structural justice to ensure that people live in just conditions and are not subject to injustices like domination, marginalization, exploitation, and oppression. In this way, institutions, systems, and individuals can provide the resources and opportunities people with mental illness need to be more resilient.

Addressing the social determinants of mental health thus requires changing the social norms and structures that create these conditions.[16] The literature on social determinants of mental health shows that these social factors constitute risk factors for mental health problems (as well as other social problems), indicating that mental health problems need to be addressed not only through a clinical approach but also through a public health approach,[17] and, I would add, a social justice approach. These risk factors must be directly addressed through social programs and structural change that improve people's living conditions, create socioeconomic security, eliminate stigma and discrimination, and ameliorate environmental conditions. Addressing these social conditions will enable us to improve people's health, both physical and mental.[18] Whether one is committed to a welfarist or a liberal view of the state, addressing the social determinants of mental health is important because it both enhances well-being and increases freedom and autonomy by giving individuals the resources they need to be able to develop and pursue their own conception of the good.

It is important to understand that the relationship between negative social factors and mental health problems is, in a vicious circle, bidirectional.[19] This is because, as addressed in chapter 2, these vulnerabilities are structurally linked and compounding, exacerbating each other. Situational vulnerabilities and mental vulnerabilities (as well as other ontological vulnerabilities) all worsen each other and add to the overall burden of vulnerability a person experiences. Just as negative social factors impact mental health, mental health also negatively impacts these social factors. Poor mental health worsens people's living conditions, making it harder to hold down jobs, receive an education, live in safe and stable housing, and be protected from adverse environmental conditions. When people have mental health challenges, they are more likely to be stigmatized, socially excluded, and discriminated against. Poor mental health makes it harder to deal with adverse childhood experiences and racism.

Since the relationship between negative social factors and poor mental health is bidirectional, addressing one of these factors helps to ameliorate other factors. Improving mental health through increased access to mental health treatment also often improves living conditions, socioeconomic conditions, and social conditions. Making people's living conditions, socioeconomic conditions, and social conditions better through social programs and structural change also tends to reduce chronic stress, thereby increasing mental health. For this reason, the project of addressing mental health must involve addressing social, socioeconomic, and environmental conditions as well. We cannot attain health, well-being, and justice in one area without attaining it in other areas as well. Because negative social, socioeconomic, and environmental conditions stem largely from structural features, addressing these requires reforming structures to be more just.

A Structural Justice Approach

A social justice approach looks at how power is distributed among individuals based on how they are socially situated. Iris Marion Young describes social justice as follows: "The matters of social justice . . . concern whether the background conditions of people's actions are fair, whether it is fair that whole categories of persons have vastly wider options and opportunities than others, how among the opportunities that some people have is the ability, through the way institutions operate, to dominate or exploit others, or benefit from their domination and exploitation."[20] Social justice is concerned with how much power and privilege some people have in relation to others based on how they are socially situated, and how benefits and burdens, and resources and opportunities, are distributed in society based on this.

One dimension of social justice is distributive justice, which looks at how resources and opportunities are distributed within a society. Enabling individuals to have secure access to what they need—including housing, employment, and healthcare—is a matter of distributive justice. As described in chapter 5, justice requires designing institutions that have as some of their duties to provide these resources in order to realize people's human rights by meeting their basic needs. Institutions have greater power and capacity than individuals and are better able to create access to resources and opportunities. The rehabilitative programs that helped Steele obtain housing, employment, and mental healthcare were fulfilling their duties of distributive justice to meet the needs of vulnerable individuals—and to fulfill their human rights.

Another aspect of social justice, which this chapter concerns, is structural justice. Structural injustice occurs when some people are positioned in such ways as to receive systematic burdens and harms due to how they are situated socially, while other people are positioned in such ways as to receive systematic benefits. When people who are burdened are dominated, exploited, marginalized, or otherwise oppressed, they experience structural injustice. Young says, "Structural injustice, then, exists when social processes put large groups of persons under systematic threat of domination or deprivation of the means to develop and exercise their capacities, at the same time that these processes enable others to dominate or to have a wide range of opportunities for developing and exercising capacities available to them."[21] When people are systematically burdened and oppressed due to how they are socially situated, allowing others to benefit from their harms, they experience structural injustice.

While Young does not clarify what kinds of "capacities" she is referring to in emphasizing the importance of developing and exercising capacities, I take her to mean whatever capacities are necessary for exercising basic human capacities such as agency and autonomy. The more opportunities that people have to develop their capacities, the wider the range of choices they are capable of making and the more options for action they have. The more options people have, the more thoroughly they can consider different values and goals. Exercising various capabilities is necessary for developing agency and autonomy.

When structures are just, they allow people adequate opportunities to exercise these capabilities. When structures are unjust, they close off opportunities for exercising capabilities and consequently block certain courses of action, impeding what possibilities people have. This decreases their agency and their capacity to value and to pursue their self-chosen ends. One of the greatest harms of structural injustice is the way that it constrains agency and autonomy. Structural justice, on the other hand, improves access to resources and opportunities, thus increasing options for people and allowing them greater choice. This enhances their agency and autonomy.

Creating access to resources and opportunities that enable options and increase choices is central to structural justice. When rehabilitative programs enabled Steele to receive housing, employment, and mental healthcare, they helped him achieve structural justice, at least in this respect. When no structures enabled this access, on the other hand— when he was homeless, unemployed, and uninsured—the private housing, employment, and healthcare systems that precluded access for people like him to their resources were subjecting him to injustice. Even institutions that are designed to meet people's needs can be unjust in how they are structured, however, when they lack mechanisms for the people whose lives they govern to be empowered. The extent to which the rehabilitative programs that helped Steele were just depends on what mechanisms they had for him to be able to exercise his agency and autonomy.

How people are situated conditions what options and constraints they have for their action. As discussed in chapter 2, some people are more vulnerable than others depending on how they are situated in relation to structures in society. People who experience social vulnerabilities, such as vulnerability to homelessness, violence, or mental illness, inhabit what Young calls a "social-structural position" that "differ[s] from persons differently situated in the range of options available to them and in the nature of the constraints on their action."[22] Whether people who are positioned as being dispositionally vulnerable to harms such as homelessness, violence, or mental illness actually experience occurrent harms depends on several factors, including their own choices and actions, luck, and the choices and actions of others.[23] After all, the choices that other people make have consequences for what kinds of choices are available to a particular person. How one is situated impacts what outcomes a person experiences as a result of other people's choices.

How people are situated socially is a relational position, where some are harmed by certain social processes while others benefit from the same processes and thus benefit at the expense of those who are harmed. People who experience structural injustice therefore experience injustice *in relation to* others who profit from their injustice. For example, economic exploitation occurs when poor people have no good options and are forced to take what options are available to them; wealthier people benefit from being able to amass wealth at the expense of poor people's options.[24] Those who profit from injustice are granted more opportunities and more options for action by the way social structures are set up, while those who experience injustice have fewer opportunities and fewer possibilities. Those who benefit from unjust structures are thus granted more agency and autonomy through that benefit, while those who are burdened have major constraints on their agency and autonomy.

Structural injustice results from the confluence of the combined actions of multiple agents, where any given action may seem to be morally innocent, but together they culminate in major harms to those who are situated in disadvantaged ways. Thus, it can appear that a given institution or individual is acting well in their circumstance, yet their action can contribute to a greater harm. Housing markets, job markets, healthcare systems, and hospitals can all appear to have just practices because some people benefit from them, but a systematic examination of the people who are harmed by these systems and institutions shows that their practices can add up to create considerable harm to certain groups of people.

People who experience social harms like homelessness, violence, and mental illness have decreased agency and autonomy due to how they are positioned in society relative to others who are positioned differently. Those who are positioned in advantageous ways profit from the same system that burdens others by gaining more choices and options through the same processes that constrain those who are disadvantaged. People who have safe and stable housing, who experience relative safety and security, and who are mentally healthy experience greater agency and autonomy within a system that burdens those who lack these advantages with more constraints on their agency and autonomy. For example, middle-class, well-educated people who own their own homes have more options for where and how they work because they have more resources they can draw upon, while people who lack advanced education and who are subject to rising apartment rents have fewer options for what kind of work they can take on.

Social structures constrain and enable possibilities, affecting people who are differently situated within the structure in different ways. Young notes that the way social structures constrain is by closing off certain options, thus blocking possibilities. But they do not do this in an intentional, direct way. Rather, this constraining happens as the result of a confluence of different agents' actions, including the actions of individuals and of institutions. She says, "Social structures do not constrain in the form of the direct coercion of some individuals over others; they constrain more indirectly and cumulatively as blocking possibilities. Part of the difficulty of seeing structures, moreover, is that we do not experience particular institutions, particular material facts, or particular rules as themselves the source of constraint; the constraint occurs through the joint action of individuals within institutions and given physical conditions as they affect our possibilities."[25]

Reduced opportunity for those who are burdened results from the cumulative effects of many different individuals' and institutions' actions. Such actions are typically not made in concert with each other, but rather they occur as discrete actions that have cumulative effects. For this reason, we cannot isolate and identify specific agents that acted badly to cause structural injustice; rather, structural injustice results as a cumulative effect of many agents' discrete actions that together enable some possibilities for people who can access them and close off others. Many of the social determinants of mental health result from structural injustices where, on their own, particular individuals and institutions seem to do nothing wrong, yet their actions taken together cause considerable harm to vulnerable people.[26]

People who benefit from structural injustice have increased resources to draw upon in their efforts to be resilient, while people who experience structural injustice have diminished resources and therefore less capability to be resilient. Young says, "What differentiates social positions is that different rules apply to people in different positions, and people in different positions have different kinds and amounts of resources available to them to mobilize in an effort to achieve their goals."[27] People in different social positions have different power, privilege, resources, and opportunities; those who have less of these do so because social rules are more restrictive for them. As a result, they have less ability to mobilize resources to advance their goals and interests. Because resilience requires drawing on various resources, people who are differently situated consequently have differing abilities to be resilient.

Addressing structural injustices improves mental health by decreasing the chronic stress people are exposed to when subject to the social determinants of mental health, while better mental health improves people's ability to live within and deal with structural injustices. Having good mental health does not itself change structural injustices, because unjust structures exist independently of the quality of individuals' mental health, but it does help people deal with their situation better because it enables people to access resources that are needed for resilience. When a person has good mental health, they have better inner resources to draw upon in dealing with various life challenges. Improving mental health thus increases people's ability to deal with structural injustices they face, while addressing structural injustice decreases the chronic stress individuals experience, thus improving people's mental health.

Institutional Response to Structural Injustice

Individuals and institutions both have duties of structural justice, which are obligations to make structures more just.[28] Because they have different capacities and power, however, the ways in which they can work on making structures more just varies. Institutions have more power to change social norms, rules, and policies, and they can influence each other by setting examples, by persuasion, and by arranging conditions to make some actions easier to do than others. Since individual action is usually less impactful (except for those who have significant power and wealth), most individuals have to work within institutions to have more of an effect. For individuals, carrying out duties of structural justice often involves playing a role within an institutional program rather than acting as an isolated agent. For this reason, it is important to focus on the institutional duties of structural injustice inherent in institutions and systems.

As discussed in chapters 2 and 5, institutions and systems structure the choices and actions people can take. They provide the conceptual tools, language, and epistemic resources that allow people to understand their situations and themselves. They make some options for action available and close off other options. They provide reasons for action that serve as motivation. In this way, they provide the context for choice, both subjectively (what people perceive as their options) and objectively (what options are actually available); they provide the context in which action occurs and supply the action with meaning and significance. In short, they enable the kind and extent of epistemic and moral agency that people can have in given situations.

A structural justice approach looks at how institutions help structure the lives of people who have mental illness, assessing the quality, resourcefulness, and justice of these institutions and advocating for reform where these institutions are impoverished or unjust. It is not only the quality of institutions that are designed to meet people's needs that must be examined, but also the quality of *all* institutions and systems with which individuals interact insofar as these institutions and systems help structure the lives of such individuals. *All* institutions and systems with which people with mental illness interact should be sufficiently resourceful and just so as to be supportive and protective. In this way, they can avoid causing the structural injustices that create the social factors that impede mental health. This enables people to get their mental health needs met without causing other kinds of harm such as creating pathogenic vulnerabilities, which institutions and systems sometimes do.

As noted in chapter 5, institutions and systems can be impoverished or resourceful, sometimes both in different areas. They can make certain resources and not others available to people based on different criteria of access. They can provide opportunities for those who qualify for those opportunities. They can also provide support, enabling people to act in ways that allow them to accomplish their goals. When they are resourceful, they provide the conditions that enable agency, autonomy, and meaning-making capacity. When they are impoverished, they can create pathogenic vulnerabilities, making people more susceptible to harm than they already are, and cause structural injustices that lead to negative social factors that imperil mental health.

Injustice can occur through impoverishment, but it can also occur through systems of domination—such as coercion, abuse, violence, or neglect—and oppression, such as exploitation, discrimination, or marginalization.[29] People who have mental illness or who are situated as mental patients are especially vulnerable to these types of harms and injustices because their social position grants them less power and privilege compared to the people operating the institutions and systems that govern their lives.

For example, psychiatric hospitals are easily the sites of domination, since they operate as what Erving Goffman called "total institutions": institutions that have as their main goal to manage people, which they accomplish by dictating nearly every aspect of a patient's life.[30] They employ strict schedules for patients, they require patients to participate in activities such as meals and group therapy with fellow patients, and they make the activities in what are normally various spheres of life (work, sleeping, eating, and leisure time) all occur in the same space so a patient no longer has boundaries between different areas of their life. Psychiatric hospitals manage people in order to promote crisis stabilization and patient and staff safety. In such a totalizing environment, acts of domination are easily normalized. Coercion, abuse, and violence are not uncommon in such institutions where staff have almost all of the power and patients have almost none.

Individuals play a role in structural justice or injustice by acting in relation to institutions. Young describes the duties of structural justice that individuals have according to a social connection model of responsibility.[31] While a liability model of responsibility looks backward at what happened to identify agents who are causally responsible for certain harmful outcomes, a social connection model examines the background conditions that are normally taken for granted to assess how just they are, and it looks forward at what changes need to occur to make them just. Rather than identifying specific agents as responsible, it recognizes that all agents that exist within social structures have forward-looking duties to change to be more just. The responsibility to make structures more just is a shared responsibility of all relevant agents that can only be discharged through collective action of multiple agents working together. Individuals thus have duties to engage in collective action with others to change structures and institutional practices to make them more just.

What actions institutions must take in order to be more just depends on the specific context of the institution and the structural conditions in which it acts. In Steele's case, there needed to be more jobs available for people like him so that he would not be vulnerable to sexual and economic exploitation. The private housing market needed to have a way for people without adequate income, like him, to be housed; the employment market needed to have a way for people with severe mental illness, and people who lacked stable housing, to obtain a job; the healthcare system needed to have a way for people without health insurance to be able to access needed healthcare. Hospitals needed to have mechanisms to avoid coercing patients and to prevent abuse and violence. All of these systems and institutions needed to have mechanisms for people like Steele to make needs claims or rights claims that would be heard, respected, and responded to.

Empowerment and Justice in Uptake

One of the ways that institutions can promote structural justice is to increase the power of the individuals whose lives they govern. When individuals have more power, they are less likely to be exploited, marginalized, dominated, coerced, or manipulated, or subject to violence or abuse. The primary way for individuals to have more power is to have more voice, to have a greater say in what happens to them so they have greater control over their circumstances. This empowerment increases resilience, because it gives individuals more options for how they can change their situation and increases agency and autonomy. Structural justice thus requires that institutions and systems have mechanisms to enable the individuals whose lives they govern to have more power.

Empowerment of disadvantaged people allows individuals to have more access to social goods, and it gives people more opportunities so they can escape the constraints imposed on them by structures that would otherwise burden them. Empowerment is thus a matter of social justice. Mechanisms that allow individuals to have more power rearrange the power differential in the social relationships between individuals and institutions. While empowerment is important for people with mental illness, who are often made powerless by their illness and by being positioned as mental patients receiving mental healthcare treatment, it is also important for *all* disadvantaged people who experience the negative social factors that contribute to poorer mental health.

Empowerment promotes resilience. It gives people more access to resources and opportunities that they can channel in trying to transform their situation or to transform themselves so they can deal with their situation better. By increasing agency and autonomy, empowerment makes it easier for people to deal with mental illness and to deal with the life challenges that can lead to poor mental health. Empowerment also transforms relationships of power so that vulnerable people are not subject to the structural injustices that create negative social factors that imperil mental health.

One way that institutions can empower the individuals whose lives they govern is to create mechanisms for individuals to share their ideas and concerns so that they will be listened to, taken seriously, and responded to appropriately. This helps address the epistemic dimensions of social vulnerability, where people are granted less credibility and less epistemic power in being recognized as legitimate participants in epistemic practices due to how they are socially situated,[32] as well as the moral dimensions of lacking power to change one's situation. With this in mind, I propose that institutions have at least two specific duties in relation to structural justice: the duty to listen to the individuals whose lives they structure, and the duty to take up individuals' ideas and concerns where relevant by being responsive to them, changing as warranted. By listening and being responsive, institutions empower individuals to have a voice that is listened to and to be able to exert some control over their circumstances.

This promotes an aspect of social justice that I call justice in uptake. Justice in uptake involves treating individuals fairly by taking their testimony seriously and being appropriately responsive to it. Justice in uptake has both an epistemic component, where individuals have to be listened to *well* and deeply in order to be accorded with the respect they deserve, treated as fully legitimate participants in shared epistemic practice; and a moral component, where institutions have to make intentional changes based on what they hear from individuals. Both institutions and individuals have duties to ensure justice in uptake, as both interpersonal interactions and institutional interactions contribute to structural (in)justice. In what follows, I explain what the two duties of justice in uptake—listening and being responsive—involve.

DUTY TO LISTEN

One important duty that institutions and individuals have is the duty to listen deeply to the ideas, reasons, needs, interests, and desires of vulnerable people. Institutions have this duty in order to empower the individuals whose lives they govern, while individuals have this duty in order to contribute to structurally just conditions and to help institutions carry out *their* duties of listening. While listening is often thought of as an interpersonal activity between an individual speaker and an individual listener, it can also be seen as an institutional activity where institutions have mechanisms to listen to and take seriously the ideas of individuals, as well as to communicate their own ideas. Both individuals and institutions have a duty to listen in order to be able to understand what the self-chosen ends and corresponding needs of a vulnerable person are to promote their autonomy and dignity and to be appropriately responsive.

Good listening treats the speaker as a legitimate participant in epistemic practices. Through listening carefully, an individual or institution regards the speaker as having credibility, as *worthy* of being listened to and taken seriously. Good listening thus helps promote epistemic justice, particularly testimonial justice, where a person's testimony is regarded as credible and taken seriously as appropriate to the circumstances.[33]

Joseph Beatty presents a traditional understanding of listening, which involves a desire to understand the person to whom one is listening, and where the purpose of listening is to try to gain that understanding. Beatty notes, "The good listener focuses her attention on the other's communication in order to understand the other's meaning or experience."[34] A person can listen for the sake of many ends, including making judgments, solving problems, morally appraising the other, or gaining approval of the other, but these are not central to the act of listening; what is central is trying to understand the other.[35]

Susan Notess objects that listening is not about achieving a specific end, such as full understanding, but about participating in the process of relationship-building.[36] Gaining understanding may be a key *motivation* to listen, but the *end* or goal of listening cannot be to achieve full understanding, as that would be an unattainable goal and is not the appropriate goal for listening. Full understanding may not be possible; it may not be possible even to have knowledge of whether one fully understands.[37] Rather, listening is "a dynamic and ongoing process"[38] involved with establishing a relationship. Listening is thus inherently relational, as it is an activity that structures the relationship between speaker and listener.

Notess describes listening as "a kind of skilful action which features throughout the fabric of our lives and structures the way we treat others."[39] For Notess, the main goal of listening is to develop a certain kind of relationship, one of uptake and responsiveness, between speaker and listener. She observes, "The core task of listening then is not the processing of speakers' *claims*, but the establishing and maintaining of such adequately open and responsive relations to *the speakers themselves*."[40] Listening is thus for the sake of relationship-building.

I think that it is fair to say that *trying to gain understanding* should be understood as an ongoing process that involves curiosity—the desire to know and understand more—and epistemic humility—the recognition that one does not have, and possibly could never have, full understanding. With humility and curiosity, a person recognizes that they will never be able to achieve the goal of *full* understanding, yet they are committed to the goal of continuously *trying to understand more* than they currently do, recognizing that no matter how much they *do* understand, they can always try to understand more. In this view, full understanding is an impossible goal, and not the appropriate goal for listening; the goal instead is *trying to achieve greater understanding* than one currently has, continually. Through this continuous pursuit of further knowledge and deeper understanding, a person also engages in the process of relationship-building through the very mechanisms involved with trying to achieve that understanding. Developing an open and responsive relationship between speaker and listener is thus a function of the goal to gain greater understanding than one already has.

Both individuals and institutions have duties to listen with the goal of trying to achieve greater understanding than they already have. This is especially the case in relation to the expression of needs, rights claims, concerns, and self-chosen ends. When vulnerable people express their needs, concerns or self-chosen ends, or make rights claims, they need to be heard properly so that the institutions and individuals who are working with them can *understand* their concerns and claims from the vulnerable person's own point of view rather than imposing needs, ends, or rights claims on them. This understanding allows institutions and individuals to be appropriately responsive, and responsive in ways that are autonomy-promoting. Only by understanding a person's situation adequately, from their own point of view, can an individual or institution intervene intentionally in ways that build agency and autonomy.

When vulnerable people express concerns or problems, or identify harms or injustices, they need to be heard properly so that individuals and institutions can understand the nature of the problem or harm and respond in an appropriate way that addresses the problem or harm. Furthermore, when vulnerable people express what their self-chosen ends are—what they value, what their goals are, what they want to achieve—institutions that work with them and individuals that provide care to them need to hear these self-chosen ends so the institution or individual can work to promote the vulnerable person's self-chosen ends rather than ends that the institution or individual imposes on them. In this way, interventions can be autonomy-promoting and care can be dignifying. Achieving greater understanding through listening is necessary for being able to respond appropriately.

In addition to being inherently relational, listening is also inherently situated. Listening can be understood as a compound act involving a set of specific practices, where different practices are undertaken in different kinds of listening, for example hearing intonations of sound from which one acquires meaning in a spoken conversation versus opening and reading text messages in a text conversation. Some of the activities involved with listening include tracking the literal meaning of communications, attending to body language and emotional tones, participating in an internal dialogue in the process of trying to make sense of a communication, positing and examining preliminary understandings and conclusions, observing pattens and connections to be made between different communications, and monitoring one's own reactions to the content and emotional context of communications.[41] We participate in these practices within particular social, political, economic, environmental, and individual contexts that shape how these practices occur.[42]

These contexts shape the expectations we have of our listening, the assumptions we make while we are listening, and the ways that we interpret meaning. We make many assumptions when we are listening about how communications are given, how they should be heard, what emotions and thought processes are involved, and what communications mean. What is left unsaid is often just as important as what is said, but more easily ignored. Speech that is left unsaid sometimes masks structural violence and oppression.[43] Justice requires that individuals and institutions listening to vulnerable people pay attention to the contexts in which people speak—or do not speak—in order to be cognizant of the power relations that structure how speech and lack of speech are performed and perceived.

Good listening requires both detachment from one's own mental states and investment and engagement with what the speaker says. In order to achieve testimonial justice, a listener must take seriously the views and experience of the speaker. This involves, in part, resisting the common tendency to be influenced by prejudices and biases that shape how the listener understands what the speaker is saying. Beatty and Notess propose different means of achieving this resistance to bias, with Beatty focusing on detachment and Notess focusing on engagement.

Beatty argues that good listening requires detachment from one's own mental states, which he defines as "reason's or intelligence's attempt to free itself from whatever is or could be an obstacle to the understanding of what is real, true, or meaningful."[44] A listener should engage in reflective distancing in order to enable "more cognitive access to the true or meaningful."[45] This involves detachment from not only the traditional ideas of emotions and passions, but also detachment from previously held reasons, motivations, judgments, reactions, and so forth; in other words, detachment from all of one's own mental states. In the context of institutional listening, this requires that mechanisms of listening to vulnerable people's needs and concerns involve detachment from institutional interests, assumptions, and tendencies in order to genuinely hear what the vulnerable person expresses.

To accomplish detachment, a person has to be self-aware of their own orientation toward the speaker and speech, for example aware of their prejudgments and emotional tendencies.[46] Self-awareness is thus necessary for good listening. In the context of institutional listening, this means that institutions must be aware of their own biases, interests, assumptions, tendencies, and norms, and be intentional about having mechanisms for listening that do not activate these. This is especially important when vulnerable people share concerns or needs related to the institution itself, such as feedback on how well something is working. Institutions must detach themselves from their own self-interest and really hear what feedback vulnerable people give, without biases, assumptions, or self-interest getting in the way.

Detachment from one's own mental states is critical for empathy. We can understand empathy here as imaginatively reconstructing the experience and perspective of the speaker from their own point of view.[47] The process of imaginatively reconstructing someone else's experience requires that we put aside our own feelings, thoughts, and experiences in order to better understand someone else's experience within their own framework of meaning, not ours. For institutional listening, this requires that institutions have mechanisms for individuals working within them to develop empathy for the vulnerable people whose lives they govern. Through detachment, individuals and institutions can better understand the person to whom they are listening.

While Beatty argues that good listening requires detachment from one's own mental states, Notess argues that good listening requires engagement with and investment in the speaker's experience and views. This involves three steps: first, that the listener makes a judgment about the importance of the speech they are hearing; second, that the listener uses this judgment of importance to determine how much effort they should put into processing the meaning of the speech; and, third, that the listener is willing to be open to persuasion.[48] In this way, they can be appropriately *responsive* to the speaker.

When a listener judges speech as unimportant, they are not motivated to put effort into processing its meaning, and they are not willing to be open to being affected by the speech. This failure in the motivational component of listening can result in *unjust* listening, where a person does not listen *well*, and not listening leads to epistemic injustice of not taking the speaker seriously. When a listener, whether an individual or an institution, regards speech as important, on the other hand, they are motivated to put effort, sometimes significant effort, into processing its meaning and participating in more relevant activities involved with listening, such as paying close attention, filling in gaps, making inferences, and seeing implications.[49] In addition, they are more willing to be open to being moved by and transformed by the speech. Notess describes listening "as involving active tasks of managing how one processes and responds to others on the basis of one's willingness to centre, elaborate on, and respond to the other person's speech."[50]

We can add a fourth step of what engagement with and investment in the speaker's experience and views involve. It requires that a listener do their best to understand the experience or situation of the individual or entity to whom they are listening and the perspective the individual or entity has based on this. Understanding the situation and perspective of the individual or entity with whom one is communicating can enhance that communication. For example, understanding the powers and limitations of an institution, as well as understanding its structure, mission, and goals, can aid a person in communicating with members of that institution whose job it is to carry out the institution's mission and goals.

Institutions and individuals interacting with vulnerable people need to practice both detachment and engagement in order to listen *well*. They need to listen to the ideas, reasons, needs, interests, desires, values, and goals of vulnerable people with the aim of trying to understand more what their experience is like and what perspectives they hold and why. The goal is not to gain full understanding, but to continuously try to understand *more*. For both individuals and institutions, detaching oneself from one's own mental states means detaching oneself from one's own perspective, worldview, and interests in order to more fully understand the perspective, worldview, and interests of the speaker. Engaging with the speaker requires judging that what the speaker says is important, putting effort into the activities involved with listening, and being open to being persuaded, and to changing one's view and action as appropriate.

Listening well requires seeking out more voices, especially of people who are particularly vulnerable and marginalized, so that one has a broader understanding of the relevant experience and issues. For institutions, this requires adopting mechanisms of seeking out the voices of vulnerable people that the institution is trying to help, as well as mechanisms of

Resources for Social Justice   177

gaining feedback. Feedback is especially important in being successful at helping the people the institution is intended to help, in order to learn how successfully the intended interventions are working; after all, interventions may have unintended consequences that the institution would otherwise be unaware of if they did not seek out feedback. When individuals and institutions listen well to vulnerable people, they also model what listening well looks like and serve as role models for vulnerable people as to how they should act as well.

Listening well also requires openness, or being willing to be persuaded, and being willing to change one's views or action if warranted. This includes being open to criticism, where one is willing to learn from the criticism in order to transform and become better. Individuals have to open their hearts to be able to be open in this way, while institutions need to adopt mechanisms not only of obtaining feedback but also of changing in response to that feedback. This kind of listening constitutes what Jonathan Lear calls the virtue of the chickadee: to listen to others with the intention of learning from them so that one may reshape oneself in relation to the given situation.[51]

DUTY TO BE RESPONSIVE

Being responsive is an important duty that both individuals and institutions have in enabling social justice. We can call this kind of justice "justice in uptake." Justice in uptake involves taking seriously the expression and needs of a speaker, affording them appropriate credibility and legitimacy, and responding to what is expressed or needed as appropriate to the context.

In a testimonial context, uptake is "a dialogical responsiveness and openness"[52] to testimony. Being responsive and open involves respecting, attending to, and empathizing with a speaker. Giving uptake well involves having a certain disposition, where one takes seriously and attends to the views of the speaker. Nancy Nyquist Potter identifies uptake as an Aristotelian virtue: a middle state between expecting certainty in speech and dismissing speech as discreditable.[53] Uptake involves regarding speech as credible and thus important, worthy of being taken seriously; it also involves taking speech seriously by paying attention to what it calls for and responding to it as needed.

Uptake can be thought of as a middle state in other ways as well. As a mean between accepting testimony at face value and dismissing it as discreditable, uptake involves engagement with testimony. In general, this means trying to attain deeper understanding; sometimes, this means interrogating testimony critically. Critical interrogation is only appropriate in some circumstances, depending on whether the default position should be to trust the speaker or to be skeptical toward them; in the right circumstances, however, it can be an important aspect of taking testimony seriously.

In addition, uptake can be understood as a middle state between regarding testimony as conclusive, a final word that closes out inquiry, and regarding testimony as so insignificant that it doesn't even begin inquiry. In this conception, the middle state involves engaging in inquiry that is open-ended, again, sometimes simply to gain deeper understanding and sometimes to interrogate critically. This active engagement should accompany a willingness to change one's view or actions if the testimony warrants it or to direct one's actions according to the testimony, where this is understood as a middle state between changing for any or no reason at all, and an unwillingness to change. This willingness to change or to have one's actions directed is what makes uptake *responsive*. Active engagement with testimony, with a willingness to change views or actions if testimony warrants it, or to direct actions as testimony suggests, are necessary components of uptake.

Uptake is important not just for testimony, but also for the sharing of ideas, suggestions, conceptual frameworks, desires, needs, interests, values, and goals. Any expression of need or concern should be taken up responsibly and responsively. Any idea or suggestion should be taken seriously, considered, and used as motivation for change if warranted. Expressions of emotion should be taken up seriously, as well, as sometimes the way a concern is voiced—for example, with anger or bitterness—matters to the content of what is voiced.[54] Ideas, suggestions, conceptual frameworks, desires, needs, interests, values, goals, and emotions should be engaged with for the sake of developing greater understanding of the speaker offering them, and sometimes critically interrogated to examine how true, useful, or important they are. Listeners should use this active engagement as a motivation for potential change.

To fail to take up ideas, suggestions, conceptual frameworks, desires, needs, interests, values, goals, or emotions responsively is to discredit and disrespect potentially vulnerable people. People have power when their voice is properly heard and responded to; vulnerable people have greater power—which they can mobilize to have more power over the situation that makes them vulnerable—when they are listened to responsively. In a community where uptake is normalized and regularized, vulnerable people more easily have justice in uptake.

Having testimony, ideas, suggestions, needs, interests, values, and goals taken up appropriately is important for people to be able to exercise epistemic agency, or participation in epistemic practices with others, as well as moral agency. Other people have to take up a person's epistemic contributions and respond to them appropriately for the contributions to be recognized as counting as legitimate epistemic practice. Other people also have to be willing to engage with and respond appropriately to a person's expression of needs, interests, desires, values, or goals for these to be recognized as contributing to moral practice. This is why epistemic and moral agency require a community: only by participating with others in a shared exchange of ideas, or action and response, does one's individual speech or action constitute epistemic or moral practice. When others take up a person's testimony, ideas, suggestions, needs, interests, desires, values, goals, or emotions, this enables the person's contribution to have an effect on the world, thus enabling their agency—and granting them power.

When testimony, ideas, suggestions, and concerns are taken up appropriately, this also aids in meaning-making. Through testimonial exchange of ideas, vulnerable people participate in the process of developing understanding and making meaning of their experience. Through this process, they can be exposed to new conceptual frameworks for understanding their experience and find new ways that their experience is significant. Being treated as fully legitimate epistemic participants whose ideas are responded to appropriately enhances understanding and meaning-making.

In addition, uptake enables autonomy. Uptake is important for being able to see oneself in the future and to conceptualize future goals and actions. When others are appropriately responsive, they can open up new possibilities that weren't available before, increasing a person's options for action and increasing what they can imagine themselves doing. Others' responsivity can help a person to be able to see possibilities that they were not previously aware of, giving them more reasons to hope for a better future. Uptake is thus important for both conceptualizing goals and enabling hope, both of which are central for successful autonomy.

Moreover, when a person shares their values and goals—their self-chosen ends, what is important to them—and others respect these ends and help the person to achieve them, this fosters autonomy by helping a person to live the life they choose. Respecting a person's ends and helping them to achieve these ends is a form of uptake. It involves listening to a person's values and goals, taking them seriously, and being willing to direct one's action accordingly to help promote them.

Uptake and responsiveness enable resilience. When institutions and individuals are responsive to a person's expression of needs, concerns, interests, values, or goals, they direct their action accordingly. This has the potential to change the situation the vulnerable person finds themselves in. When institutions and individuals are responsive, they enable the vulnerable person to whom they are responding to have some control over their situation through being able to voice their needs in a way that is heard and responded to. This control helps a person to cope with their situation more effectively by changing it, thus enabling resilience.

Listening, uptake, and responsiveness change the power dynamic between the vulnerable person and the institution or individual with whom they interact, giving more power to the vulnerable person in relation to the institution or individual. This enables the vulnerable person to have more control and autonomy in the relationship. This also grants the vulnerable person more credibility and legitimacy as an epistemic participant, increasing their epistemic power as well as their moral power. Instead of being at the mercy of the institution or individual wielding power, the vulnerable person has power that they can wield as well, through their voice. By changing the power dynamic, the actions of listening, uptake, and responsiveness help to create more just structures that govern the interactions of the vulnerable person. This helps to promote social justice.

In the context of mental illness, it can sometimes be hard for individuals with mental illness to voice their needs and concerns in a way that is heard by others. This is partly because their mental illness can diminish their credibility through mental illness stigma, and partly because mental illness symptoms can make it difficult to voice their needs and concerns in a manner that is heard and respected, that is, in a rational, controlled, and empowered way. In such a context, health advocates can play an important role in facilitating uptake and providing legitimacy and credibility to people who might not otherwise be listened to appropriately. Moreover, it is not just vulnerable individuals themselves who need to be listened to and taken seriously; their caretakers need this, too. Family members of people with mental illness, for example, are sometimes ignored or not taken seriously in healthcare contexts, but their needs and concerns also deserve uptake. Health advocates can help with facilitating caretaker uptake and enabling caretakers to have legitimacy and credibility as well.

The duties to listen and to be responsive are only one aspect of social justice. Social justice also requires other actions that change the way benefits and burdens, and resources and opportunities, are distributed in a society. But they are an important step, and one that helps improve the agency, autonomy, and resilience of vulnerable people.

Conclusion

As Steele's story demonstrates, people who are especially vulnerable due to conditions like mental illness frequently experience compounding situational vulnerabilities that exacerbate each other. Many of these vulnerabilities are due to social injustices, where structures benefit some people with power and privilege, as well as resources and opportunities, while burdening other people with constraints on these. This leads to burdened people having more limitations on their agency and autonomy and being less able to live the kind of lives they want to live. When social structures are unjust, they allow individual behavior and institutional practices to perpetuate social injustices.

Justice in uptake is one way to transform unjust power relationships to be more just. With justice in uptake, institutions and individuals have duties to listen to the vulnerable people with whom they interact and to be appropriately responsive based on what they hear. Taking seriously people's expression of ideas, suggestions, needs, concerns, desires, interests, values, goals, and emotions and responding to them accordingly gives the individuals sharing these contributions some power over their circumstances, leading to increased control, enhanced agency and autonomy, and greater resilience. Increasing vulnerable individuals' epistemic and moral agency also transforms power relationships so that people are not subject to the structural injustices that negatively impact mental health.

People who have mental illness need many kinds of support, resources, and opportunities to be successful at being resilient in the face of mental health and other life challenges. In chapters 3–6, I have examined some of the social support and inner and external resources that people need to be able to be resilient. In addition, people need opportunities to find and create meaning in their experiences. In chapter 7, I examine the value of purpose and meaning in one's life and what kinds of opportunities people need in order to achieve these.

Chapter 7

Opportunities for Meaning

Introduction

In their recovery, it was important to both Elyn Saks and Ken Steele to have opportunities to find and create meaning. One way that they did this was through participating in meaningful activity. This helped them deal with their illness and gave them purpose in their lives that made it easier to cope with suffering. In being able to pursue meaning, they were able to focus on positive areas of their life and learn and grow as individuals.

Saks's primary form of meaningful activity was work. Over and over in her memoir, she emphasizes the value of work to her life and her ability to cope with her illness. She says, "I knew that work, more than anything else I could do, would steady me."[1] Work provided her with a deep source of meaning and worth. She says, "For me, my worth was defined in and by *work*."[2]

Some of her psychiatrists recognized this and encouraged her to use it to help her. One of the doctors who worked with her when she was hospitalized as a graduate student in England encouraged her to stay in school and continue working in her program. Saks says, "Dr. Storr's subsequent recommendations were not only simple, they were in direct contradiction to those made by the doctors who four months before had suggested I leave school and be hospitalized. 'Your mind is very sick,' he said calmly, 'and just as I'd advise with a sick body, it needs a specific kind of exercise to help it heal. That means resuming the work that you love. It makes you happy, it gives you purpose, it challenges you. And so you need to stay at Oxford, in your program.'"[3] She was very happy to follow this recommendation.

Steele also identified work and meaningful activity in general as being conducive to his mental health. He notes, "Whenever I was deeply immersed in something (like my efforts to prepare for, and get, a job in the nursing home) or engaged with people I trusted, the voices lost their commanding influence on me."[4] In reading his memoir, one is struck over and over by his work ethic, his dedication to whatever job he has at the time and the hard work he put into it. Several times, he expresses as one of his goals to earn a living for himself so he could take care of himself and not have to rely on others—and also not be stuck in a hospital where others took care of him.

When he did not have a paid job (and even sometimes when he did), he sought out volunteer work to keep him busy. In Hawaii, he sought out volunteer work at the mental health center where he received services, and he winded up starting a self-help group and writing a literature review for the center in which he researched Alcoholics Anonymous and other peer support groups and wrote a paper on his research findings. He ended up writing and receiving a grant based on his research, presenting his proposal to the Hawaiian legislature.[5] Being involved with something so important significantly raised his self-esteem, self-worth, and self-respect.

Work helped him manage his voices and other mental illness symptoms so they were not as predominant in his life. When he lost one job, he notes that he became "confused, disoriented, and easy prey for the voices which told me again and again what a terrible failure I was."[6] When he was working, he was able to manage his life better and take care of himself better, which helped diminish his symptoms.

For both Saks and Steele, it was important that they make a difference in people's lives. In particular, they wanted to make a difference in the lives of people like them, people who had severe mental illness who suffered from both their illness and the social structures and systems that were intended to help them. Not only did they want to work as a way to engage in activity that was meaningful *to them*, but they also wanted to contribute to society by effecting change in the lives of others.

After Saks was hospitalized as a graduate student, she sought out volunteer work in neighboring psychiatric hospitals, because she felt that, as an insider who knew what it was like to be a patient in a psychiatric hospital, she had something special to offer to other patients. She says, "I decided I wanted to make some sort of contribution, to repay my debt to the professionals who'd taken such good care of me, hoping that in the process I might be able to help others. I believed that I understood the experience of being in a hospital for the mentally ill in a way that the staff (or at least most of the staff) might not—which logically, I thought, would make me a good volunteer."[7] In fact, her personal experience helped her connect with the patients she worked with.

As a law professor, she was also dedicated to helping make a difference in the lives of people with severe mental illness like her. She chose to specialize in law related to psychiatric disability. Her first significant publication was a note for the *Yale Law Journal*, titled "The Use of Mechanical Restraints in Psychiatric Hospitals." The Bazelon Center for Mental Health Law informed her that they had used the note to challenge the use of restraints in a Midwestern hospital. She writes of her pride in her accomplishment, "My work had made a difference. It helped another attorney and it helped patients who were no different from me. No different at all."[8] She went on to publish many more articles in this field.

Steele similarly wanted to make a difference. When he heard politicians on the radio and television wanting to remove systems that supported people with mental illness, such as SSI (Supplemental Security Income), SSD (Social Security Disability), and Medicaid, he was angered. He says of these politicians, "They demanded cutbacks in community mental health services, treatment, housing, and research. They expected us, the mentally ill, somehow to pull ourselves up by our own bootstraps. If we failed, we could wind up homeless or in jail. It mattered little to these political voices. They simply did not want our care to cost them money."[9] In reaction to these sentiments, Steele started the Mental Health Voter Empowerment Project in 1994 in New York City, increasing voter registration of people with mental illness by thousands. He wanted people with mental illness to be enfranchised so they could vote for politicians who had their interests at heart.

As a result of this work, he obtained many opportunities to work with mental health education and outreach. He participated on a panel with psychiatrists about how the clubhouse system worked, with its treatment access and day programs, work opportunities, community, and residences. He did a public service announcement for NAMI (National Alliance on Mental Illness).[10] In 1995, he started editing *New York City Voices: A Consumer Journal for Mental Health*, which then had a circulation of 2,500; he widened coverage from four pages to thirty-two pages, expanded readership (which grew to 40,000 by 2001), and publicized the Mental Health Voter Empowerment Project.[11] He created an Information and Referral Service, which he manned himself at his home, answering people's questions about everything from legal issues to treatment, giving advice for how to support people with mental illness.[12] He wrote for websites, addressed self-help organizations by sharing his personal story, and started a self-help group he ran out of his own apartment.[13] He gave public speeches to organizations, both on television and on the radio.[14] His activism landed him on the front page of the *New York Times* in 1999.[15] Through all of these efforts, Steele made a huge difference in the lives of thousands of people with mental illness.

When he began this work, he was still hearing voices and interacting with his psychosis. Yet, just as with his paid work, he found he could manage the work by focusing on what needed to be done. Even when the voices were chattering, he could focus enough attention on the work that he could momentarily ignore them. In fact, work, both paid and volunteer, was a source of solace and refuge for him. He did the bulk of his volunteer work, however, after his voices left him when he was taking Risperdal. Without his voices, he was able to experience a meaningful recovery from psychosis, and he was committed to giving back and helping others who were like him.

As we see from Steele's and Saks's stories, recovery from mental illness requires a person to pursue meaning and purpose in their life. Finding and creating meaning allows a person to cope with mental health and other life challenges, and this requires opportunities to engage in the pursuit of meaning. Meaning-making consists of assigning significance, purpose, meaning, and salience in experience, events, objects, and people (including oneself); it also involves making sense of experiences, events, the world, and oneself. It is one of the core functions of being human, a function that must be preserved and exercised for a person to be successfully resilient.

One important aspect of recovery from mental illness involves making a life of meaning for oneself despite one's illness. Recovery is not necessarily about getting better—many people with mental illness do not experience a linear recovery that ends in getting better[16]—but rather about being able to manage one's illness so that one can have a meaningful life that is not dictated by illness. The search for meaning is a key component of this.

Recovery from mental illness involves several aspects.[17] Clinical recovery consists of diminished symptoms and improved functionality.[18] While remission is not always possible, diminished symptoms can be a key goal because this helps individuals focus on and develop other areas of their life. Functional recovery is often tied to clinical recovery because it is made possible by a diminishment of symptoms; it involves being able to function well in various areas of one's life, including social relationships, social interactions, employment, and education. Clinical recovery is also tied to physical health. To achieve physical health recovery, a person pursues a healthy lifestyle that includes eating well, sleeping well, and exercising.

In addition to clinical, functional, and physical health recovery, people with mental illness also engage with various aspects of personal recovery. According to William Anthony, personal recovery "involves the development of new meaning and purposes in one's life as one grows beyond the catastrophic effects of mental illness."[19] Patricia Deegan describes recovery as a process or journey of meaning-making and working on goals one sets for oneself, not necessarily culminating in a particular ending or final accomplishment. She says, "Recovery is a process, not an end point or a destination. Recovery is an attitude, a way of approaching the day and the challenges I face. Being in recovery means that I know that I have certain limitations and things I can't do. But rather than letting these limitations be an occasion for despair and giving up, I have learned that in knowing what I can't do, I also open upon the possibilities of all the things I can do."[20] For both Anthony and Deegan, recovery involves developing autonomous agency and meaning in one's life so that one can make a good life for oneself despite having illness.

Some aspects of personal recovery are existential, where a person develops agency and empowerment, hope, self-concept, self-care, self-efficacy, and spiritual well-being.[21] Meaning-making and pursuit of meaningful activity are critical to developing these capacities. Participating in meaningful activity also supports functional recovery, where a person participates in activities involved in various life domains, and it can decrease symptoms by enabling people to focus on different areas of their life. Other aspects of personal recovery are social, where a person develops stronger relationships with the people around them as well as connection to a community and a sense of belonging, which leads to increased agency and responsibility as a person gains the ability to be accountable to others.[22] Social engagement is central for this aspect of creating meaning. As discussed in chapter 4 in the context of social support, social engagement also improves functioning and physical health and can decrease symptoms, thus impacting other areas of recovery.

In order to be able to work on their recovery, people with mental illness need to have opportunities to find and create meaning and purpose. This enables people to be resilient in the face of adversity: to examine their difficulties, change their situation where they can, and adjust to and accept their situation when it is beyond their control. In enabling resilience, meaning and purpose also enable recovery. The ability to cope with illness and suffering allows the pursuit of a life of meaning that is not dictated by illness.

Meaning

Meaning and purpose foster resilience in many ways. Having a sense of purpose in one's actions and experiences provides a profound sense of fulfillment and satisfaction, which aids self-esteem and self-efficacy. Seeing meaning in what happens to a person and in what they do gives a person strength, motivation, and courage to deal with whatever comes their way and opens the door to creativity, equanimity, mindfulness, and problem-solving. In addition, having meaning helps a person interact with others in more positive and productive ways, resulting in more and better social engagement, which can lead to increased social support, social networking, and belonging. When a person has meaning in their life, they are better able to draw on their inner resources as well as better able to access the social resources they need for resilience. Meaning and purpose make it possible to acquire and develop the skills, virtues, mindset, and resources needed for resilience.

Meaning not only helps provide tools for resilience, but it also makes it easier to bear difficulties, as having meaning and purpose in one's life allows a person to endure what could otherwise be difficult to bear. Viktor Frankl famously quotes the philosopher Friedrich Nietzsche as saying, "He who has a *why* to live for can bear almost any *how*."[23] When a person experiences significant stress that appears pointless and meaningless, this easily puts them in a state of despair. When the significant stress appears to serve some purpose, however, this makes a person less despairing and more able to deal with it. Understanding a broader context in which suffering occurs can help give suffering some meaning.

The stress itself does not have to be meaningful for a person to be motivated by meaning and purpose, however. Even if the stress itself does not appear to have any sort of purpose, simply having meaning in other areas of one's life can make the stress easier to bear. When a person experiences meaning in areas of their life such as family, friendships, work, school, and other meaningful activities and relationships, they are able to focus on those areas more and derive some pleasure and fulfillment from them. As a result, they give less (negative) attention to the significant stress they are experiencing, allowing them to deal with it more easily. Studies show that being reminded of what is meaningful decreases negative thinking about an event.[24] Being able to focus one's attention selectively on what is valuable is an important strategy for creating resilience.[25]

Meaning is relative to the person and particular to the experience in any given moment. Frankl notes that there is not a single, general, abstract meaning to life, but rather a constant search and experience of meaning that varies continuously depending on what is going on in a person's life.[26] He states, "Everyone's task [to seek meaning] is as unique as is his specific opportunity to implement it."[27] In fact, only the person themselves can determine what meaning an experience holds; no one else can do it for them. He argues, "This [search for] meaning is unique and specific in that it must and can be fulfilled by him alone; only then does it achieve a significance which will satisfy his own *will* to meaning."[28]

The meaning that a person experiences in a given moment provides motivation to act. This is why finding meaning in some area of one's life can make it easier to bear difficulties in an unrelated area: the meaning provides motivation to endure what is difficult instead of giving up or giving in to the suffering. Meaning provides motivation to pursue what is meaningful and to endure what can appear pointless, for a greater or alternative good.

Meaning also provides pleasure, satisfaction, and fulfillment. A person feels more pleasure in their life, and experiences satisfaction and fulfillment, when they have meaning in certain areas of their life. The fulfillment is experienced directly when the person can focus on the area of their life in which they find meaning, but it also bleeds into other areas: a person can feel indirect fulfillment when they know in a recess of their mind that there is meaning in some area, even if they have to focus, in the moment, on a different area of their life where they may find less or no meaning (such as a place in their life where they experience suffering).

Meaning enables the transformation of self and situation that is involved with resilience, and it enables a person not simply to cope with what happens to them but also to grow from the experience. As studies of natural disaster victims show, having meaning in one's life increases resilience, allowing a person to cope with disaster in productive ways, and enables people to grow from adversity.[29] When a person has meaning in their life, they are better able to access and exercise the inner resources required for resilience, and better able to access necessary external resources. Being connected to what is important in life helps a person to be more grounded; to have better motivation and willpower; to have stronger self-concept, self-esteem, and self-efficacy; to be more connected to other people; and to be more successful at accomplishing goals. These all help a person access the support and resources necessary for resilience.

Meaning can take many forms. Some ways of attaining meaning are through mindfulness (living in the present moment) and through savoring moments, whether from the past (through memory), present (through mindfulness), or future (through anticipation).[30] Gratitude helps a person appreciate positive aspects of their lives, while performing acts of kindness for others helps a person feel like they make a difference in the lives of others.[31] Appreciation of art and beauty, spending time in nature, and pursuing religious or spiritual experiences are common sources of meaning.[32] Escaping into one's own mind and memory, which belongs ultimately only to oneself, can help provide the meaning that enables resilience,[33] as can using humor to cope.[34]

Gillian A. King, Tamzin Cathers, Elizabeth G. Brown, and Elizabeth MacKinnon identify three primary sources of meaning, which can be encapsulated by the ideas of belonging, understanding, and doing.[35] What these authors understand as "belonging," I understand more generally as social engagement. People gain significant meaning from interpersonal relationships and social interactions, which provide support, connection, and a sense of belonging. Understanding one's experiences and situation more deeply, and understanding oneself, others, and the world all provide another source of meaning. This meaning-making is an epistemic process of making sense of the world, oneself, one's experiences and actions, and others by fitting these within a broader context of meaning that makes them intelligible. In addition, people attain meaning from determining what is valuable, setting goals for themselves, and working toward achieving these goals. In other words, the ability to pursue meaningful activity involved with exercising autonomy and agency provides a third place where people create meaning.

These three sources of meaning point us to three kinds of opportunities that people need in order to be able to find and create meaning. People need opportunities for social interactions and developing social relationships; they need opportunities to understand and make sense of their experiences and actions, as well as themselves, the world, and other people, more deeply; and they need opportunities to engage in activities that are meaningful to them, creating and working toward goals that they value. Thus, they need the world to create openings for them to have social interactions, to help them reframe their experiences in meaningful ways, and to find places where they can work to achieve the kind of life they want for themselves.

Social Engagement

First, vulnerable people who are in need of meaning in order to bolster their resilience require opportunities for social interactions and for developing social relationships. Through this, they can gain a sense of belonging, social support, and recognition that supports self-esteem. In chapter 3, I discussed the importance of social support in fostering resilience; belonging and recognition are also key.

Both Saks and Steele write about social interactions that were meaningful to them by making a difference in how they saw the world and how they were able to respond to events, and social relationships that helped them develop their identity and agency, and their capacity for self-care and self-efficacy. Saks writes fondly of friendships that she valued tremendously,[36] and Steele describes acts of kindness and aid by the people around him that enabled him to see the world and himself differently, and to engage in the world in a more meaningful way that was not governed by his voices.[37] Social interactions and social relationships were central to their ability to be resilient and to make a life of meaning for themselves.

Social relationships that provide a sense of belonging are a significant source of meaning and motivation. People are willing to work through problems and endure what is unavoidable for the sake of others whom they care about and for the sake of receiving care from others. Social interactions in general provide a sense of belonging, where people find even small interactions meaningful because of someone's kindness, for example. The meaningfulness of small interactions adds up to a sense of meaning in one's general interactions with the world, making acting in the world feel purposeful and valuable. Such meaning helps foster people's sense that they are capable of problem-solving and enduring suffering.

In addition, recognition by others promotes meaning by enhancing a person's self-concept, increasing their self-esteem and self-worth, and even improving self-efficacy.[38] Since people's identities are relational, how other people see a person affects who the person is and how they see themselves.[39] Other people's recognition of a person helps the person formulate a conception of who they are, defining their self-concept. When a person is recognized by others as a valued member of their community, they gain self-esteem and self-worth as they learn to recognize their own value through the eyes of others. When they interact with others who accept them as part of their moral and epistemic community, they are able to have an effect on the world that matters, impacting the others with whom they are interacting, thus enhancing their self-efficacy.

Social engagement is critical for developing and exercising agency. As I have written about elsewhere, social engagement enables the development and exercise of many epistemic and moral skills and virtues that are required for epistemic and moral agency.[40] Social interaction is necessary for many capacities associated with epistemic agency, including intelligibility (shared meaning), shared understanding of the world, responsiveness to evidential norms, self-understanding, and epistemic trust. It is also necessary for many capacities associated with moral agency, including cognitive skills, emotional capacities, and valuation capacities. In addition, social interaction is necessary for the development of many aspects of moral agency and integrity, including autonomy, moral identity, recognition by others as a member of a shared moral (and epistemic) community, and responsibility.

All of these capacities and aspects of moral and epistemic agency are important for being able to mobilize resources in the process of resilience. Being able to change or accept and adjust to one's situation requires the exercise of both epistemic and moral agency. A person has to interact with others as a knower and a moral agent to understand their situation in its complexity and to problem-solve, implement strategies, redirect their energies, and simply endure. In enabling resilience, these capacities and aspects of moral agency also enable a person to establish and live out a life of meaning that is not overcome by illness.

In a virtuous circle, meaning and social engagement are bidirectional: meaning helps increase social engagement and social support, and social support, belonging, and recognition provide an important source of meaning. Social interactions and relationships help provide a sense of belonging by connecting people to a community, giving them a sense of meaning, and enabling them to gain a social network that can be a crucial source of social support. At the same time, having a sense of meaning in at least some areas of one's life makes it easier for a person to interact well with others: to interact in meaningful ways that are positive and productive. Meaning and social engagement each support each other, so that increasing one also increases the other.

Meaning-Making

Both Saks and Steele engage in a variety of activities involved with meaning-making, especially by sharing their stories through written, published narratives that are read by a wide audience. In constructing a narrative, they make sense of their experience by imposing order on it through narrative structure and genre. In sharing their story with the public, they enable other people to learn from and connect with their experience.

Steele recognizes that his story brought people hope. As he started telling his story to public audiences, he realized, "To my surprise . . . people wanted to hear more about my personal recovery story—probably because I had met and conquered obstacles faced by many in the audience, and I gave them hope."[41] His success at overcoming his demons—and his ability to cope with the suffering he endured for decades—is inspiring to others. Some of the meaning that Steele finds and shows us in his story is the hope that things can get better.

Saks recognizes that through her story she is teaching others what having a severe mental illness can be like. She concludes her memoir with some life lessons, which I quoted in the introduction to this book: "What I rather wish to say is that the humanity we all share is more important than the mental illness we may not. With proper treatment, someone who is mentally ill can lead a full and rich life. What makes life wonderful—good friends, a satisfying job, loving relationships—is just as valuable for those of us who struggle with schizophrenia as for anyone else."[42] She also has pointed advice for people who have severe mental illness like her: "If you are a person with mental illness, the challenge is to find the life that's right for you."[43] Some of the meaning that Saks finds in her experience is the need to live a full, rich life of one's own choosing.

Meaning-making is a process of assigning meaning to experience and action based on one's beliefs, goals, values, and feelings.[44] Beliefs about oneself, the world, and other people help shape what kind of meaning one gives to these. Values are principles used to govern one's behavior, influencing how a person acts to try to attain their goals. Goals provide motivation and purpose, as well as standards for assessing behavior; working toward goals provides a source of self-esteem and self-worth, as well as self-efficacy. Having meaning in one's life is in part affective, as it involves a subjective sense that life, or at least aspects of life, are meaningful.[45]

Meaning-making involves contextualizing experience. It is a process of fitting one's experience within a larger frame of meaning that includes one's beliefs, values, goals, and feelings. Crystal Park and Jeanne Slattery argue that the overarching goal of meaning-making is to achieve consistency between one's experiences and one's beliefs, values, goals, and feelings.[46] Beliefs and values that help a person cope with adversity provide a framework for making sense of adversity. For example, the belief that life goes on and that one will recover from adversity helps give a framework for accepting what is uncontrollable about adversity and for enduring what is painful to get through the pain.[47] The belief that one can learn from suffering and grow as an individual can help a person view something about their situation that is positive, enabling them to endure the suffering involved for the sake of some other good. The value of trying to find some good in every situation can help a person focus on positives and not get too overwhelmed by negative aspects of their situation.

When a person's experience and their framework of meaning do not cohere, the goal of consistency requires that one has to change in relation to the other. Thus, making sense of a person's experience can involve either changing their beliefs, values, goals, and feelings to accommodate the experience, or changing their appraisal of the experience to make it fit within their meaning framework. Both options can be valuable; which option is preferable depends on the context of the situation.

Changing one's beliefs, values, goals, and feelings can be very difficult, as these are often deeply rooted. But sometimes people have transformative experiences that challenge the way they see the world and that invite them into new ways of understanding the world. Being open to changing one's meaning framework can be a resourceful way of accommodating challenging experiences and can create opportunities for new meaning and consequently new growth. For example, a person with mental illness may have deep-rooted beliefs that they will always be sick and can never get better, but seeing other sick people recover can challenge that belief, inviting them to open their mind to the possibility that they could get better.

Sometimes people start with positive beliefs and values that turn negative as a result of experience. For example, a person may have a deep-rooted belief that the world is essentially good; yet, when something terrible happens to them, this experience can challenge that belief, leading them to revise their meaning system to include a belief that there is evil in the world and perhaps a value of vengeance to "get even" with whatever/whomever is seen as the cause of this evil. This kind of transformation of one's meaning framework happens commonly in response to adversity yet is more harmful than helpful, leading to cynicism and despair rather than optimism and hope. This change in one's mindset can make it harder for a person to access inner resources needed for resilience, as cynicism and despair often make it harder for a person to exercise creativity, problem-solving skills, and perseverance.

To develop resilience, people suffering from adversity need help and guidance in changing their meaning framework in positive and productive ways that help them access and exercise their inner resources, as well as enable them to access external support and resources. The person whose experience leads them to change their beliefs and values to believe that there is evil in the world, and that they are a victim of it, may need help seeing that their particular experience is not necessarily indicative of a generalizable metaphysical worldview. In response, they might modify their beliefs and values so that they believe that neither good nor bad is intrinsic to the world, but that people can get harmed through various events and actions, and that vengeance does not solve problems.

To change their beliefs and values in positive and productive ways, vulnerable people often need the help of others to guide them in seeing the world differently. For people with mental illness, therapists play a pivotal role in this, guiding people to see the world in more realistic ways that help a person deal with and perhaps grow from adversity rather than succumbing to cynicism and despair. One of the central roles of therapy is to help clients shape their beliefs and values to be more positive and productive, enhancing the person's flourishing rather than diminishing it.

Alternatively, a person might retain their beliefs and values but change their goals and feelings by reappraising their situation. Cognitive reappraisal involves reconsidering a situation in a different light. It can involve seeing aspects of the situation one did not see before and focusing on some aspects as salient while ignoring others as irrelevant or unhelpful. With cognitive reappraisal, a person may be able to appreciate some good that came out of the experience of adversity or see the experience as a learning opportunity. This can change the feelings a person has toward the situation, such as reducing despair and inspiring hope or finding meaning in the situation.

Cognitive reappraisal can even increase control over a situation. By allowing a person to see the situation in a different light, reappraisal can enable creativity and problem-solving skills that help a person to change the situation in some way. This increases self-efficacy and self-esteem, as well, which increases positive feelings toward the situation, including hope and meaning.

Cognitive reappraisal is a process of reframing, or what Crystal Park and Jeanne Slattery call "recounting" or "restorying" experiences of adversity.[48] This reframing places the experience in a different meaning context that helps make sense of the experience without requiring a person to change their beliefs or values. Allison Troy and Iris Mauss note that cognitive reappraisal "involves reframing an emotionally negative situation in a more positive way to decrease feelings of negative emotion" as well as to increase positive emotions.[49] As a form of emotion regulation,[50] cognitive reappraisal helps a person deal with the emotional reactions they have to events in a way that helps rather than hinders their flourishing.

Reappraising a situation can help a person adjust to a situation that they have little or no control over so that they can endure it and deal with it with less suffering. As Susanne Schwager and Klaus Rothermund note, "Reappraising a situation often involves a reorganization of goals and an adjustment of personal standards and aspiration levels to a given situation."[51] Reappraising thus often involves changing one's feelings about the situation as well as changing the goals and expectations one has in relation to the situation. In fact, adjusting expectations and goals is a central way for people to be able to assimilate themselves to a situation that they have little or no control over.

Of course, for cognitive reappraisal to work, a person must endorse it as an adequate description of the situation.[52] If it does not adequately explain the facts of the situation as the person sees them, it will not serve as an alternative way to consider the situation and will have little use. Only an adequate explanation can serve as a legitimate option that one can endorse.

Here again, therapists play an important role in guiding clients to see their situations in alternative, helpful ways. Often a person cannot see their situation differently without the help of someone else who can offer a different perspective. While the perspective of many other people—including friends and family—can be helpful, the perspective of a therapist can be particularly helpful as they are trained to help individuals see their issues in ways that are productive to their mental health.

As we see from Steele's and Saks's memoirs, cognitive appraisal is often done in the context of constructing a narrative about one's experience. Narrative construction does not have to be formalized; the informal stories we all tell ourselves about ourselves constitute personal narratives about experience, too. Both informal and formal narratives help us understand ourselves and evaluate and make sense of our situation better.

Recounting a story of one's experience involves putting order on events so they are made intelligible. People with mental illness often experience their symptoms and suffering as a chaotic jumble of events, or a searing intensity of experience that isolates it from other experience. Chaotic or atomistic experience can lead a person to feel a disunity of self, an inability to integrate experience into their self-concept, personal identity, and sense of agency. Constructing a narrative of experience locates experience in a larger framework of meaning, connected to other events and experiences in a way that makes sense of them. This allows a person to integrate experience into a larger understanding of the course of their lives, allowing them to incorporate the experience into their self-concept, identity, and sense of agency.

Putting order on events is a way of exerting control over them. A person may not be able to change how events occur, but they can determine what meaning the events have, and this is a form of control. Through this process, they can exercise agency and resilience. People with mental illness often feel like their condition and situation is out of their control, and this can cause great despair. Being able to put order on their experience allows them some control over how the experience affects them and makes hope possible.

People with mental illness often create personal narratives that explain, as best they can, what happened to them, how, and why. Frequently this situates their experience in time, with a beginning that explains how their illness started, a middle that describes the experience of illness and suffering itself, and an open-ended conclusion that points to where they might go in their lives and that will only be filled out as they continue to live their lives. The beginning often identifies possible causal factors that led to the illness, and the ending often identifies goals and values the person wants to pursue or is in the midst of pursuing. The middle typically points to beliefs, desires, and motivations the person holds, and how their experience shaped these. Identifying these aspects of meaning is a way of anchoring the details of one's story within a meaning framework that makes sense of it.

Personal narratives often fit standard genres of illness narratives, such as restitution narratives (where a person gets sick and then gets better), chaos narratives (where a person experiences a lack of coherence in their story, cannot identify causal factors, and/or cannot lead to a tidy conclusion), or quest narratives (where a person gains something positive from their experience).[53] Other narrative genres include escape (recovery from illness or leaving the mental health system), enlightenment (where growth occurs), or endurance (simply living with illness and suffering even as a person is unable to control or change it).[54] Narrative arcs sometimes focus on being sick, coping, or getting better.[55] Narrative genres and arcs are different forms that structure the story of a person's experience as a way of imposing control over it. Through narrative genres and arcs, people find and create meaning in their experience.

Personal narratives are often situated within a broader master narrative about mental illness, such as a biomedical or psychosocial narrative of mental illness that explains experience in biomedical or psychosocial terms.[56] People have a tendency to adopt master narratives as frameworks to understand the details of their experience in ways that makes sense culturally. Biomedical and psychosocial narratives are the dominant master narratives in Western culture, but alternative narratives that explain illness as dangerous gifts, or in spiritual terms, can also serve as master narratives that frame a person's individual experience.[57]

As noted in chapter 2, sometimes people adopt dominant master narratives that frame illness in terms of what Şerife Tekin calls "DSM culture," a way of looking at illness experience entirely in terms of symptoms or diagnostic criteria based on the *Diagnostic and Statistical Manual*.[58] This can lead to impoverished self-insight, narrow self-concept, and diminished self-efficacy. This narrow understanding of experience can make a person see themselves primarily in terms of problems or deficits, leading to diminished self-esteem and a narrow self-understanding. The focus on problems and deficits can make it hard for a person to see—and thus access and exercise—their strengths and inner resources, limiting what control they have over their lives, leading to lower self-efficacy. By not recognizing the self as a relational self whose identity is partly constituted by relationships with others, and whose ability to deal with problems partly comes from the support and resources that others can provide, this diminished self-insight can prevent people from accessing the support and resources they need to be resilient.[59]

To avoid these problems, narratives must be resourceful, helping a person to understand the many dimensions of their selfhood[60] and to recognize and build upon the support and resources to which they have access that they can mobilize in their efforts at resilience.[61] Again, therapists play an important role here in helping individuals to understand themselves and their experiences in a richer, more complex way that does not reduce to symptoms. Therapists can guide individuals to recognize the assets they have and to build upon them so they can mobilize them in their recovery.

Cognitive reappraisal and constructing a narrative are examples of epistemic agency, where a person acts in their capacity as a knower to find or create meaning and knowledge. When they construct narratives of their experience, people assign meaning to aspects of their experience as they impose order on it. In explaining their experience, they articulate motivations, beliefs, desires, values, and goals. These aspects of meaning frame how they understand what happened to them and how they felt, thought, and acted in response.

People naturally want to understand their experience better, and they often construct narratives automatically—not necessarily writing them down, and not always conveyed to other people, but in their minds as they make sense of what happened to them. This desire to understand one's experience is an aspect of the virtue of conscientiousness, of trying to pursue truth.[62] When people with mental illness construct narratives of their experience, they act as epistemic agents who are epistemically virtuous insofar as they are pursuing truth.

People can be better or worse at pursuing truth, depending on how accurate and adequate their explanations are; explanations of experience that reflect self-deception are not successfully conscientious, even though the person is engaged in the act of trying to make sense of their experience. Explanations can be more or less true depending on how well they fit the facts of the situation, as determined intersubjectively through consultation with others. Sharing one's narrative with others is a way of testing the reality of the narrative by seeing if one's personal narrative fits the way others understand the person's experience as well.

Sharing one's narrative with others formalizes it so it is not simply a relatively inchoate story one tells to oneself. Formalizing narratives by writing them down or telling them to others makes them more real to a person and strengthens a person's understanding of their motivations, beliefs, desires, values, and goals. This firming up of a person's motivations, beliefs, desires, values, and goals can be helpful when these are productive, enabling the person to flourish, but it can be harmful when these are predominantly negative or when they hinder flourishing. For example, establishing a paranoid belief that other people are "out to get" a person does not help them flourish. Formalizing a narrative is best done under the guidance of a therapist who can guide a person to understand their motivations, beliefs, desires, values, and goals in ways that are productive, or who can guide a person to examine these carefully to assess their value to the person's self-concept and self-understanding.

People's narratives about their experience can change as they acquire new ways of understanding their experience, new values and goals, and new beliefs. The story arc and the meaning framework that anchors and shapes the story can each change in relation to changes in the other. Thus, when a person engages in cognitive reappraisal, they may revise their narratives of their experience based on their meaning framework, or they may shift their meaning framework based on their self-understanding and the narrative that underlies this. Both narrative and meaning framework are dynamic and permeable, open to change and revision; in fact, both are constantly revised as a person goes through life, acquires new experiences to which they react, and develops new self-concepts based on their experience. Meaning-making is a continuous process of making sense of our ongoing experiences.

Constructing a narrative about mental illness experience not only helps a person understand what happened to them but also gives them direction in how they ought to live. Through narrative construction, a person can reassess values and goals and face the difficult existential questions of how they ought to live given the illness they have. They may need to adjust their expectations and goals for themselves to take into account the limitations their illness brings. At the same time, they may learn to recognize new abilities and inner resources they may have as a result of dealing with their illness. This reassessment can help them deal with the uncertainty and indeterminism of their illness, giving them some direction of how to live a life with which they can be satisfied, given the unavoidable constraints of their illness.

People thus need opportunities to create narratives in order to develop self-understanding as well as contribute to the shared meaning we have with others. This requires accessing mental health treatment, especially therapy, which plays a pivotal role in cognitive reappraisal and narrative construction. Psychotherapy interventions have in fact been demonstrated to improve people's sense of meaning and purpose.[63] Some specific therapies are especially good at fostering meaning; for example, Acceptance and Commitment Therapy in particular promotes meaning in people who have schizophrenia.[64] Having the opportunity to pursue cognitive reappraisal and narrative construction *well* in the process of meaning-making requires having the opportunity to participate in therapy, which in turn requires having adequate mental healthcare resources provided by a responsive state that takes care of its citizens.

The need for meaning-making in vulnerable people also requires that institutions create opportunities for individuals to construct and share their story through various venues. This benefits not only the individual who shares their story, but also the institution—and other people—who can learn from their experience. These efforts should include opportunities to revise one's story over time in relation to new events and new ways of understanding experience. In this way, the meaning of mental illness experience can be understood, shared, and proliferated.

MEANINGFUL ACTIVITY

A third way that people find and create meaning is through engaging in meaningful activity, especially activity that contributes something of value to society. For many people, engaging in meaningful activity involves working for a wage, but it can also include activities such as education, volunteer work, caretaking, making art, and sharing one's story with others. Saks and Steele each engaged in many different types of meaningful activities such as these. As discussed in the beginning of this chapter, Saks and Steele both found meaning in wanting to make a difference to others, and they found ways of doing this that were unique to them.

Meaningful activity can be purely personal, performed for its own sake, such as regular exercise, making art for oneself, gardening, or journaling; or it can contribute to society such as by helping others, producing a good or service that is valued by others, or impacting others emotionally. Certain personal pursuits have been demonstrated in studies to increase meaning in people, including yoga,[65] mindfulness exercises,[66] and religious or spiritual activity.[67] However, all activities that a person finds meaningful increase a person's sense of meaning and purpose.

Engaging in meaningful activity requires that a person has access to external resources that enable the person to engage in different kinds of activities, including employment opportunities, educational opportunities, and opportunities for volunteering, caretaking, making art, and storytelling. In order to make these activities accessible to people with mental illness, this means that society must make jobs available to people with mental illness, that society must widen educational opportunities for vulnerable people, and that society must create openings in a variety of areas where people with mental illness can engage in meaningful activity.

In order to build resilience, people must have opportunities to live the kinds of lives they want to live and participate in the kinds of activities they find meaningful. They must have their basic needs met so they can focus their attention and energies on other areas of their life that they find fulfilling. They must have reliable housing that offers stability and safety, and they must have access to jobs and education that provide a livelihood. In addition, they must have access to healthcare that enables them to be well enough to enjoy their opportunities. Moreover, they must not be subject to structural injustices that divert their energies, as I discussed in chapter 6. In short, society must see itself as a responsive state, as I discussed in chapter 5: responsive to the needs of individuals, and promoting justice and empowerment, so individuals can live the kinds of lives they want to live.

Engaging in meaningful activity is valuable for many reasons. Meaningful activity such as work enables personal development of various kinds. Depending on the nature of the activity, a person can grow intellectually, socially, physically, emotionally, and spiritually as a result of engaging in the activity. Meaningful activities give people a sense of purpose, an outlet for creativity, and a place to meet their physical, intellectual, emotional, and spiritual needs.[68] Meaningful activities enable people to live the kinds of lives they choose for themselves as well as enable resilience.

Through work and other meaningful activity, a person can develop skills and attitudes that help them be successful in their roles, leading to a sense of competence and self-efficacy. Having a sense of competence can increase a person's self-esteem, self-worth, and confidence in themselves. This can lead to significant self-growth[69] as well as make it easier to work toward maintaining mental wellness.[70] Since mental illness is often associated with a stereotype of incompetence, where a person is assumed to have a lack of practical wisdom and judgment, impeding their ability to take care of themselves,[71] developing competence through work can be a very valuable way of countering stereotypes and resisting self-stigma. In raising a person's self-esteem and confidence in themselves, competence can also increase their ability to envision positive future outcomes for themselves, thus increasing their ability to hope.

Meaningful activities that involve fulfilling roles and expectations, such as paid work, volunteer work, and caretaking give people a sense of responsibility. Occupations such as these involve performing specific tasks attached to the role involved with the work. As people doing these types of work try to live up to the expectations associated with the roles they inhabit, they develop a desire to meet those expectations and a sense of responsibility for themselves that can be dignifying. People with mental illness are often assumed to be too incompetent to be able to be responsible for much (including themselves), and, as a consequence, often have lower expectations demanded of them.[72] Being able to carry out responsibilities associated with work or caretaking helps counter this stereotype, showing others that it is appropriate to have higher expectations of them, and that they can be successful in meeting those expectations.

Contrary to many theorists who write about work[73], meaningful activities such as work do not need to involve a high degree of control or autonomy to be meaningful. Having control and flexibility over the work a person engages in is indeed one source of meaningfulness. But it is not the only source. Performing tasks that are expected of a person inhabiting a certain role *well* is another source of meaningfulness. So is learning new skills and capacities. Even rote, tedious work can be meaningful in these ways. Having the opportunity to interact with others can be another source of meaningfulness. Any activity can be meaningful under certain conditions, and high control or autonomy, while helpful, is not necessary for meaningfulness.

Engaging in meaningful activities provides structure to a person's life, giving them something specific to do at certain parts of the day and making their lives seem more manageable.[74] For many people with severe mental illness, a lack of structure increases their symptoms and decreases their self-esteem; many people with severe mental illness identify the primary source of their despair as boredom and unemployment, not psychotic symptoms.[75] Having activities to be involved with helps direct a person's attention, focus, and energy in the effort to produce something (a good or service) that is valuable. Having something specific to do at specific times of the day makes a person feel more organized and worthy, decreasing mental illness symptoms.

Meaningful activities like paid or volunteer work, education, caretaking, making art, gardening, yoga, religious activity, and storytelling are goal-directed, meaning they are aimed at achieving something. Some of the ends to be achieved include whatever good or service is produced through work; meeting people's needs through caretaking; becoming educated and acquiring skills or capacities that are helpful in life and sometimes specific jobs; increasing mindfulness and spiritual well-being; creating a product like art, narratives, or a garden. In being directed at some end, meaningful activity provides people with purpose.

It is not only the fact that the activity is goal-directed that is purposeful, however. Meaningful activity is activity that a person can do while being fully engaged in the work. It directs the person's focus, attention, energy, and effort, so that a person's conscious mental states are absorbed in the work. Being engaged in meaningful activity can put a person in a state of flow, or engaged attention, where they are so immersed in what they are doing that they do not pay attention to the passing of time; they are simply acting.[76] The purpose of meaningful activity is both to accomplish the end of the activity, and to be fully engaged in the process.

Meaningful activity is a source of interest, provides variety of experience, provides motivation, and enables autonomous agency. When people have meaningful activities, they set goals for themselves in relation to the activities, and they work on trying to achieve those goals. Meaningful activity is thus a place where people exercise agency and autonomy: determining what is good in relation to the activity and setting ends that they then put effort into trying to realize. People develop motivation in relation to the activity, being motivated to try to attain the goals they set, such as fulfilling expectations and doing a job well done. This provides interest, as well as a desirable form of experience that is different from simply experiencing mental illness symptoms.

In addition, meaningful activity can be an important place for social interaction, providing people with purpose in an additional way. Severe mental illness easily causes social isolation, where a person withdraws socially, in part due to mental illness symptoms that make it hard to be around people, and in part due to a fear of being stigmatized.[77] When people do certain types of activities, such as certain types of paid or volunteer work, caretaking, or getting an education, they naturally interact with other people in the course of their activity. They may have colleagues, fellow students, or people with whom they are caring to work; they may have a supervisor who oversees and evaluates their work. This social interaction is crucial for a person with mental illness to develop and exercise their agency, as well as provide meaning and purpose.

Activities where a person produces a good or service that is valuable to others help the person gain recognition by others as a contributing member to the community.[78] Recognition by others enhances a person's moral identity as a moral agent participating in shared practices with others in the same community. When a person is recognized by others, this often leads to others respecting the person, which can in turn lead to increased self-respect and self-esteem.[79]

As a place where people can exercise their agency and autonomy, meaningful activity plays an important role in enabling people to live a good life according to a liberal framework. In a liberal democratic and capitalist society that is designed to maximize people's ability to live according to their conception of the good (within limits), meaningful activity such as work provides an avenue for people to pursue their conception of the good life.[80] Through meaningful activity such as work, people can exercise some control over managing aspects of their life and directing their life to go the way they want.[81]

This ability to pursue one's conception of the good life through meaningful activity such as work provides a basis for respect by others and self-respect. In a liberal framework, self-respect is predicated on the belief that one's life plan or conception of the good is valuable and worthy of pursuing, and the belief that one can have success in their pursuit of it.[82] Meaningful activity is itself part of a person's conception of the good, where they are engaged in activity that they believe to be valuable, at least to themselves, and perhaps also to others. In addition, meaningful activity can allow a person to pursue other aspects of their conception of a good life, especially when it is paid work that provides them with financial means to do other things they find valuable.[83] In a liberal society, meaningful activity is a key determinant of self-respect, because it is one of the main ways that people pursue their conception of the good and carry out their life plans.[84]

People with mental illness tend to struggle with self-respect for many reasons. The impairments caused by their mental illness can lead them to feel like they have diminished competence, which can decrease their confidence in themselves. Internalization of stigma that views people with mental illness as incompetent and that regards mental illness as something that will progressively worsen over time further decrease people's confidence in themselves and self-esteem. People with mental illness often feel like they have little control over their experience and over what happens in their lives, feeling like they have major constraints on their agency. They sometimes struggle to identify what is valuable and worth pursuing, making it hard to set ends or goals for themselves and hard to identify something to strive for, thus diminishing their autonomy. When they also have lower standards of living, difficulties acquiring safe and stable housing, and loneliness due to social isolation, this impacts their self-perception and further diminishes their self-esteem and self-worth.[85] People with mental illness are in great need of the self-respect that engaging in meaningful activity affords.

Because of the value of meaningful activity in people's lives, it is of utmost importance for society to provide opportunities for people with mental illness to engage in various kinds of meaningful activities, including paid employment but also activities like volunteering, caretaking, getting an education, making art, pursuing spiritual activity, personal hobbies, and sharing one's story. It is the responsibility of the responsive state to provide these opportunities as some of the external resources that it is obligated to provide to people with mental illness in order for them to be resilient. Moreover, it is the responsibility of institutions specifically tasked with providing these opportunities—such as various employers, educational facilities, venues for art and storytelling, and nonprofit organizations that work with mentally ill people—to provide access to these opportunities specifically for people with mental illness. People with mental illness require these external resources to help them be resilient.

Conclusion

Recovery from mental illness requires creating a life of meaning. Through meaning, people can draw on inner resources and access external resources that enable them to be resilient in the face of adversity. Having meaning in one's life allows a person to cope with difficulties, giving them motivation and willpower to change what they have control over and to endure what is unavoidable, and giving them the inner resources to be able to do this. It also makes accessing external resources easier, enabling people to mobilize the resources necessary for resilience.

In order to be able to create a life of meaning, people need opportunities to find and construct meaning. Three significant sources of meaning are social engagement, meaning-making, and engaging in meaningful activity. Opportunities to participate in social interactions and to develop social relationships give people the ability to care for and be cared for by others, and enable social support, recognition, and a sense of belonging. Opportunities to participate in meaning-making allow people to engage in epistemic activities such as cognitive reappraisal and narrative construction that help them make sense of their experience by fitting their experience into larger frameworks of meaning. Opportunities to engage in meaningful activities such as work, hobbies, caretaking, and making a difference in the lives of others enable people to work toward self-chosen goals through activity that fully engages them. External resources such as those necessary to get one's basic needs met, including housing, jobs, education, and healthcare, are required for a person to engage in such opportunities successfully. Through these resources and opportunities, a person can create a life of meaning for themselves.

Since people who have mental illness experience constraints on their agency that make social engagement, meaning-making, and participating in meaningful activity difficult, they are in special need of having these opportunities made available to them. In a responsive state, institutions should be tasked with creating these kinds of opportunities specifically for vulnerable people such as those with mental illness. In this way, society can support people with mental illness to be able to create a life of meaning for themselves.

Saks and Steele each took advantage of the opportunities that were available to them to create lives of meaning. Each of them developed their own conception of the good life and found ways of pursuing this despite their limitations. Their success at forging a good life for themselves, despite significant obstacles, is the reason why they are my heroes.

Conclusion

Ken Steele and Elyn Saks are heroes of mine because they made a meaningful life for themselves despite suffering from severe mental illness. When I was struggling with psychosis, I found their stories inspiring because they showed me that it was possible for things to get better, which gave me hope. They showed me that even when a person experiences mental illness that devastates one's ability to function and to exercise basic human capacities, it was still possible for the person to learn how to reacquire these capacities, manage their illness, and have a fulfilling life.

Moreover, part of what they did to create meaning in their life was to make a difference in the lives of others. Wanting to affect others positively is an admirable trait and reflects an ethical desire to "give back" after one has received help from others. When Steele and Saks wanted to "give back," or more properly to "pay it forward," by helping others in need after they had been helped, they were embodying the reciprocity of care that Sarah Clark Miller identified, as discussed in chapter 4.

In chapter 2, I noted that vulnerability can sometimes be understood more broadly than susceptibility to harm, instead as an openness to being affected by another or by an experience or situation. Being affected by others or by an experience or situation is being vulnerable not only to risk of harm but also to change in ways that could be positive and even momentous. The desire to make a difference in the lives of others is a way of affecting others by responding to their vulnerability or openness positively. Saks and Steele both were affected by others and affected others. In being open to treatment and recovery, Steele and Saks were open to change, willing to be affected by others and by their situation. In wanting to make a difference, they were responding to the openness of others, meeting others where they were and trying to create openings and opportunities so that others had more options.

By trying to make a difference in the lives of others, Steele and Saks were trying to help people have more agency and autonomy in their lives and more power over their situation. In this way, they were exercising care that was dignifying, attending to other people's needs in a way that supported these others in pursuing their own self-chosen ends. In doing this, Steele and Saks were ethical exemplars, models of what we all should be doing: caring for others by helping them to pursue their own self-chosen ends. The particular ways that they tried to make a difference to others were their own ways of embodying what this care could look like.

Steele and Saks thus not only were the recipients of care when they were in need of the help of others, but they also found ways of giving care to others. I am humbled by Steele's and Saks's actions, and I consider them role models for enacting the kind of power I would like to have. This includes power over my own situation, where I could change aspects of my situation and learn to adapt to other aspects of my situation that are outside my control, and power in helping to make a difference by attending to others' needs.

After all, like Steele and Saks, I don't want to be defined by the intense neediness and dependency I have when I am sick, beholden to others because of the severe constraints on my agency and autonomy due to my illness; I want to be an autonomous agent who can decide for myself how I want to be in the world and work toward my self-chosen goals. Rather than being defined by my illness and put in a position of subjugation, I want to have a say over what happens to me and have the power to have an effect on the world that matters. Like Steele and Saks, I want to be an agent, directing the course of my life in the way that I choose.

Steele and Saks were able to be autonomous agents, living the kind of life they wanted to live, given their constraints, because they were able to summon enough inner resources and take advantage of what resources, support, and opportunities they had, in order to be able to make the changes necessary to cope with their mental health challenges and grow from their experiences. They were able to recover from their illness by learning to manage their illness and live a meaningful life despite their illness. In other words, they developed the resilience needed to cope with their mental health struggles so they were not defined by or dominated by their illness.

Many factors enabled Steele and Saks to be able to recover from their mental illness. These include getting their basic needs met; having access to good mental healthcare treatment; receiving services from systems and institutions designed to help them; being treated justly by individuals, institutions, and systems; having the support of friends and/ or family; developing the inner resources such as hope, problem-solving capacity, learning capacity, courage, and flexibility that enable resilience; and finding and creating meaning in their experience and in the world around them. As we saw from the examination in this book, all of these factors necessarily have a social context, where people learn to be resilient by observing and interacting with others; where people receive care, support, and protection from others; and where institutions provide the various resources and opportunities that enable resilience. Individuals can only be resilient in the context of a society that enables them to be so.

In my own recovery from psychosis, many factors contributed to my ability to finally be resilient and recover after struggling with psychosis for two years. Because of how I am socially situated, I had certain privileges that made resilience easier. Like Saks, I come from a middle-class family that has supported me in every way possible, including supporting my education and career. I also have a family of my own, including a dear husband of over twenty years, and two teenage daughters, who give me much meaning and purpose in my life. Like Saks, I have a professional job (as a professor) that is fulfilling and meaningful and is also flexible enough in many ways to accommodate my psychiatric disability. Like both Steele and Saks, I have received good mental healthcare treatment that has successfully reduced my symptoms and enabled me to function. I don't have to worry about getting my basic needs met; I own my own home, and I do not have to worry where my next meal is coming from. Nor am I subject to any significant structural injustices. Moreover, I have friends, family, and colleagues who support me and provide care and protection for me in a variety of ways.

What I did not have, during the time I was struggling with psychosis, was the inner resources that I needed to be resilient. Over the course of my treatment, I had to develop these so I could employ them. While I was sick, I felt like I had lost a lot of agency and autonomy; there was a lot that I felt I couldn't do. Anything outside my daily routine was stressful and overwhelming; I could not navigate my way through novel situations. Problems seemed insurmountable. Feeling overwhelmed by my circumstances, I lost competence in a lot of areas. Feeling impotent and stuck, I lost self-efficacy, as well as confidence in myself. I did not trust myself to be able to handle different situations. My psychosis fundamentally disempowered me.

Through intensive inpatient and outpatient therapy, I learned how to acquire some of the skills and dispositions I needed to be able to cope with my mental illness. In particular, in my IOP (intensive outpatient program) group, I learned mindfulness techniques and distress tolerance, which helped me gain equanimity and an attitude of willingness. I learned to accept my situation instead of fighting against it and found freedom in that acceptance. The therapist in my IOP group encouraged us to adopt an attitude of curiosity toward our situation to help us develop some distance from our distress; although I never mastered this, I can see how useful it would be to have.

With my therapist's help and guidance, I practiced problem-solving skills and learned how to be more creative, flexible, courageous, open to learning (such as learning how to use new technologies), and open to novel situations. In reducing my symptoms, medication helped me to have more autonomy competency. As I became more skilled, I developed more confidence in myself and my ability to deal with different situations and to cope with my mental health and other life challenges. Normally, I have very good perseverance, but I had to learn how to channel this quality so that I would not give up on myself, not feel stuck, and not believe that I would never get better. I had to change my beliefs to learn to believe in the possibility that I could get better, and I had to have the perseverance to keep working on my recovery even when it felt hopeless. My therapist helped me to reevaluate such beliefs, and he even helped me to develop hope.

I did not learn these skills, virtues, and attitudes in a vacuum. Even outside the context of mental health treatment, I had a lot of help; it was only in relation to others that I acquired these traits. I observed what other people, such as my husband, did and tried to emulate them. Noting that other people could do certain things that felt very hard to me, I thought that if they could do it, it might be possible for me to do it, too. Inspired by stories of other people who had recovered from severe mental illness, I looked up to them as role models and strived to be like them. They gave me courage and helped me to feel more confident in myself, which helped my self-efficacy and sense of power.

Having good, effective mental healthcare treatment was critical to my recovery. I would not be where I am today if not for medication and therapy. Having health insurance that paid for this treatment, and a job that afforded me the health insurance, was essential. So was being part of a society where I could look up to people as role models, learn from others, and practice these skills and virtues in my interactions with others. Having my basic needs met and not being subject to significant structural injustices was also crucial. Living in a society where institutions are tasked with aiding and protecting vulnerable people such as those with mental illness, and where individuals willingly take on roles of caring for and protecting the vulnerable, was vital. Having significant relationships and a meaningful job was also valuable.

In light of the critiques that the concept of resilience tends to be too individualistic (explored in chapter 1), one might wonder why resilience is a concept we should hold on to rather than jettison. I believe that resilience is a useful concept to retain because the idea of positive adaptation to difficult circumstances is a useful concept for understanding how one should deal with adversity. However, the nature of this positive adaptation and the social context required for it to be achieved must be developed adequately for the concept to be useful. My definition of resilience—as the capacity to mobilize adequate resources, support, and opportunities effectively to cope with adversity and challenges in a way that increases core capacities of a human being (namely agency, autonomy, and meaning-making) in order to enable functioning and flourishing—situates the concept of resilience in a social context, thus moving away from the idea of resilience as chiefly a trait of individuals. I believe that this concept usefully captures something important about the way we should deal with adversity and challenges: by mobilizing available social resources, support, and opportunities that must be supplied adequately by social institutions so that individuals can achieve the positive adaptation that allows a person to move on in their life and not be overwhelmed by their challenges.

Everyone needs resilience to be able to deal with life challenges that come their way. People who have mental illness, who are especially vulnerable to harms caused and exacerbated by their illness, have special need of resilience in order to cope with their illness and the harms it brings. Mental health is a basic need that is required for basic human capacities including agency, autonomy, and meaning-making; finding ways of coping with mental health challenges is necessary to exercise these human capacities. With resilience, people with mental illness can live a meaningful life of their own choosing that is not dictated by or heavily constrained by their illness.

As this book has shown, resilience has a necessary social context in which people can only be resilient when the right social conditions exist. Society, and the institutions it charges with this responsibility, have the obligation to meet vulnerable people's basic needs and protect them from harm and injustices, including structural injustices that contribute to mental health problems. Individuals have the responsibility to provide care and protection to vulnerable people so that those who are vulnerable can strengthen their agency and autonomy and live lives of their own choosing. Society must also provide vulnerable people with opportunities to find and create meaning. In addition, vulnerable people need social interactions and relationships that allow them to learn and exercise the inner resources needed for resilience. In order to be resilient, therefore, people need the resources, support, and opportunities provided by individuals and institutions within society that enable resilience.

Notes

Introduction

1. Elyn R. Saks, *The Center Cannot Hold: My Journey through Madness* (New York: Hyperion, 2007), 336.
2. Ken Steele and Claire Berman, *The Day the Voices Stopped: A Memoir of Madness and Hope* (New York: Basic Books, 2001), 252.
3. I chronicled my story of experiencing psychosis, being a mental patient, and undergoing recovery in Abigail Gosselin, *Mental Patient: Psychiatric Ethics from a Patient's Perspective* (Cambridge, MA: MIT Press, 2022).

Chapter 1: Enabling Mental Health Resilience

1. Saks, *The Center Cannot Hold*, 200.
2. Saks, *The Center Cannot Hold*, 182.
3. Saks, *The Center Cannot Hold*, 245.
4. Steele and Berman, *The Day the Voices Stopped*, 174.
5. Steele and Berman, *The Day the Voices Stopped*, 191.
6. Saks, *The Center Cannot Hold*, 183.
7. Steele and Berman, *The Day the Voices Stopped*, 200.
8. Steele and Berman, *The Day the Voices Stopped*, 105.
9. Steele and Berman, *The Day the Voices Stopped*, 115.
10. Morley D. Glicken, *Learning from Resilient People: Lessons We Can Apply to Counseling and Psychotherapy* (Thousand Oaks, CA: Sage, 2006), 4–5; Steven M. Southwick and Dennis S. Charney, *Resilience: The Science of Mastering Life's Greatest Challenges*, 2nd edition (Cambridge: Cambridge University Press, 2018), 8. See also William Throop's definition of adversity as bouncing back while retaining identity and function, as discussed later in this chapter. William M. Throop, "Frugality and Resilience: A Pragmatist Meditation," in *Pragmatist and*

American Philosophical Perspectives on Resilience, ed. Kelly A. Parker and Heather E. Keith (Lanham, MD: Lexington Books, 2020), 62.

11. Kelly A. Parker, "Introduction: Resilience as a Philosophical Concept," in *Pragmatist and American Philosophical Perspectives on Resilience*, ed. Kelly A. Parker and Heather E. Keith (Lanham, MD: Lexington Books, 2020), ix.

12. Mianna Lotz, "Vulnerability and Resilience: A Critical Nexus," *Theoretical Medicine and Bioethics: Philosophy of Medical Research and Practice* 37, no. 1 (February 2016): 49.

13. Alex J. Zautra, John Stuart Hall, and Kate E. Murray, "Resilience: A New Definition of Health for People and Communities," in *Handbook of Adult Resilience*, ed. John W. Reich, Alex J. Zautra, and John Stuart Hall (New York: Guilford Press, 2010), 7.

14. Quoted in Parker, "Introduction," ix.

15. Brian Walker and David Salt, *Resilience Practice: Building Capacity to Absorb Disturbance and Maintain Function* (Washington, DC: Island Press, 2012), 3.

16. Throop, "Frugality and Resilience," 62.

17. Perhaps elements of moral character—that is, a person's moral traits—might need to stay the same in order for a person to be the same person, but their personality and character can change considerably. Nina Strohminger and Shaun Nichols, "The Essential Moral Self," *Cognition* 131 (2014): 159–171.

18. Andrew Zolli and Ann Marie Healy, *Resilience: Why Things Bounce Back* (New York: Free Press, 2012), 7.

19. Zolli and Healy, *Resilience*, 8.

20. Parker, "Introduction," xi.

21. Parker, "Introduction," ix.

22. John D. Mayer and Michael A. Faber, "Personal Intelligence and Resilience: Recovery in the Shadow of Broken Consciousness," in *Handbook of Adult Resilience*, ed. John W. Reich, Alex J. Zautra, and John Stuart Hall (New York: Guilford Press, 2010), 95.

23. Kim Lützén and Béatrice Ewalds-Kvist, "Moral Distress and Its Interconnection with Moral Sensitivity and Moral Resilience: Viewed from the Philosophy of Viktor E. Frankl," *Bioethical Inquiry* 10 (2013): 317–324.

24. Zautra, Hall, and Murray, "Resilience," 6.

25. Throop, "Frugality and Resilience," 63.

26. John W. Reich, Alex J. Zautra, and John Stuart Hall, "Preface," in *Handbook of Adult Resilience*, ed. John W. Reich, Alex J. Zautra, and John Stuart Hall (New York: Guilford Press, 2010), xi.

27. Reich, Zautra, and Hall, "Preface," xii. See also the definition of resilience as successful adaptation in Zautra, Hall, and Murray, "Resilience," 4.

28. Anthony D. Ong, C. S. Bergeman, and Sy-Miin Chow, "Positive Emotions as a Basic Building Block of Resilience in Adulthood," in *Handbook of Adult*

Resilience, ed. John W. Reich, Alex J. Zautra, and John Stuart Hall (New York: Guilford Press, 2010), 82.

29. Reich, Zautra, and Hall, "Preface," xii.

30. Shannon Sullivan describes knowledge as transactional with experience, agency, and identity; I regard agency, autonomy, and meaning-making as transactional with each other, each co-constituting the other. Shannon Sullivan, *Living Across and Through Skins: Transactional Bodies, Pragmatism, and Feminism* (Bloomington, IN: Indianapolis University Press), 133–156. See discussion in Abigail Gosselin, *Humanizing Mental Illness: Enhancing Agency through Social Interaction* (Montreal: McGill-Queen's University Press, 2021), 115.

31. Of course, people can only develop these core capacities, and the resilient behaviors that enhance them, to the extent that they have some voluntary control over the relevant actions. I make these claims within the context of a voluntarist rather than deterministic understanding of human behavior.

32. Lotz, "Vulnerability and Resilience," 50 (italics original).

33. Lotz, "Vulnerability and Resilience," 50.

34. Kelly A. Parker and Daniel J. Brunson, "Catastrophe and the Beloved Community: Resources for Resilience in Josiah Royce and Martin Luther King, Jr.," in *Pragmatist and American Philosophical Perspectives on Resilience*, ed. Kelly A. Parker and Heather E. Keith (Lanham, MD: Lexington Books, 2020), 38.

35. Zautra, Hall, and Murray, "Resilience," 6–7.

36. Southwick and Charney, *Resilience*.

37. Parker and Brunson, "Catastrophe and the Beloved Community," 38–39.

38. Katie Aubrecht, "The New Vocabulary of Resilience and the Governance of University Student Life," *Studies in Social Justice* 6, no. 1 (2012): 68.

39. Martin Huth, "The Dialectics of Vulnerability: Can We Produce or Exacerbate Vulnerability by Emphasizing It as a Normative Category?," *Philosophy Today* 64, no. 3 (Summer 2020): 561.

40. David Harper and Ewen Speed, "Uncovering Recovery: The Resistible Rise of Recovery and Resilience," *Studies in Social Justice* 6, no. 1 (2012): 12.

41. Harper and Speed, "Uncovering Recovery," 12.

42. Individuals do not always appreciate the help institutions give them, even when they are designed expressly for this purpose. As Hanna Pickard explains, some people with personality disorders may not respond well to the social institutions, such as hospitals and outpatient clinics, that are designed to aid in their recovery; for such people, more specific strategies, such as holding detached blame (which involves the cognitive component of blame but not the affective component that includes the "sting" and entitlement of blame), may be necessary. Hanna Pickard, "Responsibility without Blame: Empathy and the Effective Treatment of Personality Disorder," *Philosophy, Psychiatry, & Psychology* 18, no. 3 (September 2011): 209–224.

43. Harper and Speed, "Uncovering Recovery," 13–14.
44. Aubrecht, "The New Vocabulary of Resilience and the Governance of University Student Life," 68; Alison Howell and Jijian Voronka, "Introduction: The Politics of Resilience and Recovery in Mental Health Care," *Studies in Social Justice* 6, no. 1 (2012): 4–5; Harper and Speed, "Uncovering Recovery," 14–15.
45. Howell and Voronka, "Introduction," 4–5.
46. Aubrecht, "The New Vocabulary of Resilience and the Governance of University Student Life," 71.
47. Aubrecht, "The New Vocabulary of Resilience and the Governance of University Student Life," 72.
48. Parker and Brunson, "Catastrophe and the Beloved Community," 39.

Chapter 2: Vulnerabilities of Mental Illness

1. Saks, *The Center Cannot Hold*, 168–169.
2. Saks, *The Center Cannot Hold*, 168 (italics original).
3. "Homelessness and Housing," Substance Abuse and Mental Health Services Administration, accessed August 8, 2022, https://www.samhsa.gov/homelessness-housing.
4. According to the Bureau of Justice Statistics, people who have serious mental illness comprise 45 percent of federal prison inmates, 56 percent of state prison inmates, and 64 percent of inmates in jails. Doris J. James and Lauren E. Glaze, "Mental Health Problems of Prison and Jail Inmates," Bureau of Justice Statistics NCJ 213600, September 6, 2006, accessed August 8, 2022, https://bjs.ojp.gov/library/publications/mental-health-problems-prison-and-jail-inmates.

Over 350,000 inmates in US prisons and jails have serious mental illness; this is more than ten times the number of people who are in psychiatric hospitals. Darrell Steinberg, David Mills, and Michael Romero, "When Did Prisons Become Acceptable Mental Health Care Facilities?," Stanford Law School Three Strikes Project, February 9, 2015, accessed August 8, 2022, https://law.stanford.edu/wp-content/uploads/sites/default/files/publication/863745/doc/slspublic/Report_v12.pdf.
5. Steele and Berman, *The Day the Voices Stopped*.
6. Steele and Berman, *The Day the Voices Stopped*, ix.
7. Steele and Berman, *The Day the Voices Stopped*, 116–117.
8. Rob Whitley and Benjamin F. Henwood, "Life, Liberty, and the Pursuit of Happiness: Reframing Inequities Experienced by People with Severe Mental Illness," *Psychiatric Rehabilitation Journal* 37, no. 1 (2014): 68–70.

A different study indicates that although approximately two-thirds of people with severe mental illness express a desire to work, they have an employment rate of only 15 percent. Annalee Johnson-Kwochka, Gary R. Bond, Deborah R. Becker, Robert E. Drake, and Mary Ann Greene, "Prevalence and Quality of

Individual Placement and Support (IPS) Supported Employment in the United States," *Administration and Policy in Mental Health and Mental Health Services Research* 44 (2017): 311–319.

9. Alison Luciano and Ellen Meara, "Employment Status of People with Mental Illness: National Survey Data from 2009 and 2010," *Psychiatric Services* 65, no. 10 (October 2014): 1201–1209.

10. Guy A. Boysen and Raina A. Isaacs, "Perceptions of People with Mental Illness as Sexually Exploitable," *Evolutionary Behavioral Sciences* 16, no. 1 (2022): 38–52.

11. Guy A. Boysen, Erika L. Axtell, Abigail G. Kishimoto, and Breanna L. Sampo, "Generalized Perceptions of People with Mental Illness as Exploitable," *Evolutionary Behavioral Sciences* (2021): http://dx.doi.org/10.1037/ebs0000267.

12. Verena Rossa-Roccor, Peter Schmid, and Tilman Steinert, "Victimization of People with Severe Mental Illness outside and within the Mental Health Care System: Results on Prevalence and Risk Factors from a Multicenter Study," *Frontiers in Psychiatry* 11 (2020): https://doi.org/10.3389/fpsyt.2020.563860.

13. Elizabeth Pienkos, Anne Giersch, Marie Hansen, Clara Humpston, Simon McCarthy-Jones, Aaron Mishara, Barnaby Nelson, Sohee Park, Andrea Raballo, Rajiv Sharma, Neil Thomas, and Cherise Rosen, "Hallucinations beyond Voices: A Conceptual Review of the Phenomenology of Altered Perception in Psychosis," *Schizophrenia Bulletin* 45, suppl. no. 1 (2019): S72. See also Richard P. Bentall, *Madness Explained: Psychosis and Human Nature* (New York: Penguin, 2003), 477–484.

14. Saks, *The Center Cannot Hold*, 193.

15. Steele, *The Day the Voices Stopped*, 95.

16. Gosselin, *Humanizing Mental Illness*.

17. Andrea Fiorillo and Norman Sartorius, "Mortality Gap and Physical Comorbidity of People with Severe Mental Disorders: The Public Health Scandal," *Annals of General Psychiatry* 20, Article 52 (2021), accessed October 4, 2023, https://annals-general-psychiatry.biomedcentral.com/articles/10.1186/s12991-021-00374-y.

18. Pamela Sue Anderson, Sabina Lovibond, and A. W. Moore, "Towards a New Philosophical Imaginary," *Angelaki: Journal of the Theoretical Humanities* 25, no. 1–2 (2020): 12; Roxana Baiasu, "The Openness of Vulnerability and Resilience," *Angelaki: Journal of the Theoretical Humanities* 25, no. 1–2 (2020): 254–264; Erinn C. Gilson, *The Ethics of Vulnerability: A Feminist Analysis of Social Life and Practice* (New York: Routledge, 2014), 2.

19. Catriona Mackenzie, Wendy Rogers, and Susan Dodds, "What Is Vulnerability, and Why Does It Matter for Moral Theory?," in *Vulnerability: New Essays in Ethics and Feminist Philosophy*, ed. Catriona Mackenzie, Wendy Rogers, and Susan Dodds (New York: Oxford University Press, 2014), 1–31. See also Gilson, *The Ethics of Vulnerability*, 37; and Lotz, "Vulnerability and Resilience," 45–59.

20. Martha Albertson Fineman, "The Vulnerable Subject: Anchoring Equality in the Human Condition," *Yale Journal of Law and Feminism* 20, no. 1 (2008): 8–10.

21. Bryan S. Turner, *Vulnerability and Human Rights* (University Park: Pennsylvania State University Press, 2006), 9.

22. Fineman, "The Vulnerable Subject," 8.

23. Fineman, "The Vulnerable Subject," 9.

24. Fineman, "The Vulnerable Subject," 11.

25. Consider the way different aspects of personhood—and different ways we can be embodied and en-minded—can be unified or disunified within a person. Steve Matthews, "Blaming Agents and Excusing Persons: The Case of DID," *Philosophy, Psychiatry, & Psychology* 10, no. 2 (June 2003): 169–174.

26. Judith Butler, "Rethinking Vulnerability and Resistance," in *Vulnerability in Resistance*, ed. Judith Butler, Zeynep Gambetti, and Leticia Sabsay (Durham, NC: Duke University Press, 2016), 12–27.

27. Butler, "Rethinking Vulnerability and Resistance," 24.

28. For more information about how dominant or "master" narratives shape individual experience, see Hilde Lindemann Nelson, *Damaged Identities, Narrative Repair* (Ithaca, NY: Cornell University Press, 2001); Moin Syed and Kate C. McLean, "Master Narrative Methodology: A Primer for Conducting Structural-Psychological Research," *Cultural Diversity and Ethnic Minority Psychology* 29, no. 1 (2023): 53–63; Moin Syed and Kate C. McLean, "Who Gets to Live the Good Life? Master Narratives, Identity, and Well-Being within a Marginalizing Society," *Journal of Research in Personality* 100 (2022): 1–7, Article 104285.

29. Şerife Tekin, "Self-Insight in the Time of Mood Disorders: After the Diagnosis, beyond the Treatment," *Philosophy, Psychiatry, & Psychology* 21, no. 2 (June 2014): 139–155.

30. Patrick W. Corrigan and Petra Kleinlein, "The Impact of Mental Illness Stigma," in *On the Stigma of Mental Illness: Practical Strategies for Research and Social Change*, ed. Patrick W. Corrigan (Washington, DC: American Psychological Association, 2005), 25–26; Maria Veroniki Karidi, Costas N. Stefanis, Christos Theleritis, Maria Tzedaki, Andreas D. Rabavilas, and Nicholas C. Stefanis, "Perceived Social Stigma, Self-Concept, and Self-Stigmatization of Patient with Schizophrenia," *Comprehensive Psychiatry* 51 (2010): 19–30.

31. Butler, "Rethinking Vulnerability and Resistance," 21.

32. Butler, "Rethinking Vulnerability and Resistance," 21.

33. Turner, *Vulnerability and Human Rights*, 26.

34. Turner, *Vulnerability and Human Rights*, 28.

35. Jonathan Lear, *Radical Hope: Ethics in the Face of Cultural Devastation* (Cambridge, MA: Harvard University Press, 2006), 120 (italics original).

36. Lear, *Radical Hope*.

37. Miranda Fricker, *Epistemic Injustice: Power and the Ethics of Knowing* (Oxford: Oxford University Press, 2007).

38. Gosselin, *Humanizing Mental Illness*.

39. Gosselin, *Mental Patient*.
40. Turner, *Vulnerability and Human Rights*, 27.
41. Fineman, "The Vulnerable Subject," 10.
42. Lotz, "Vulnerability and Resilience," 47.
43. Mackenzie, Rogers, and Dodds, "What Is Vulnerability, and Why Does It Matter for Moral Theory?," 6.
44. John J. McGrath, "Variations in the Incidence of Schizophrenia: Data versus Dogma," *Schizophrenia Bulletin* 32, no. 1 (January 2006): 195–197.
45. Adolf Meyer, *Psychobiology* (Springfield, IL: Charles C. Thomas, 1957).
46. Catriona Mackenzie, "The Importance of Relational Autonomy and Capabilities for an Ethics of Vulnerability," in *Vulnerability: New Essays in Ethics and Feminist Philosophy*, ed. Catriona Mackenzie, Wendy Rogers, and Susan Dodds (New York: Oxford University Press, 2014), 39.
47. Susan Dodds, "Dependence, Care, and Vulnerability," in *Vulnerability: New Essays in Ethics and Feminist Philosophy*, ed. Catriona Mackenzie, Wendy Rogers, and Susan Dodds (New York: Oxford University Press, 2014), 189; Mackenzie, "The Importance of Relational Autonomy and Capabilities for an Ethics of Vulnerability," 46.
48. Huth, "The Dialectics of Vulnerability," 570.
49. Dodds, "Dependence, Care, and Vulnerability," 192.
50. Steele and Berman, *The Day the Voices Stopped*, 175–176.
51. Dodds, "Dependence, Care, and Vulnerability," 199.
52. Mackenzie, "The Importance of Relational Autonomy and Capabilities for an Ethics of Vulnerability," 46.
53. Steve Matthews and Jeanette Kennett, "Respecting Agency in Dementia Care: When Should Truthfulness Give Way?," *Journal of Applied Philosophy* 39, no. 1 (February 2022): 117–131.
54. Mackenzie, "The Importance of Relational Autonomy and Capabilities for an Ethics of Vulnerability," 47.
55. Mackenzie, "The Importance of Relational Autonomy and Capabilities for an Ethics of Vulnerability," 46.
56. Lisa Dodson, *The Moral Underground: How Ordinary Americans Subvert an Unfair Economy* (New York: New Press, 2011).
57. Hanna Pickard, "The Puzzle of Addiction," in *The Routledge Handbook of Philosophy and Science of Addiction*, ed. H. Pickard and S. H. Ahmed (London: Routledge, 2018), 9–22; Hanna Pickard, "What We're Not Talking about When We Talk about Addiction," *Hastings Center Report* 50, no. 4 (2020): 37–46.
58. Steve Matthews, Robyn Dwyer, and Anke Snoek, "Stigma and Self-Stigma in Addiction," *Bioethical Inquiry* 14 (2017): 275–286.
59. Gosselin, *Humanizing Mental Illness*.
60. Abigail Gosselin, "'A Useful Resource': Work Justice for People with Mental Illness," in *Peaceful Approaches for a More Peaceful World*, ed. Sanjay Lal (Leiden: Brill, 2022), 239–269. Of course, work is not necessary for engaging

in meaningful activity that contributes to society; other forms of activity can fulfill this function as well, as I explain in chapter 7. Nonetheless, work is one valuable way that many people in society do engage in meaningful activity, and it is a means that should be available to more people with mental illness, as they have just as much of a need to engage in this type of activity as other people do.

61. Wendy Rogers, "Vulnerability and Bioethics," in *Vulnerability: New Essays in Ethics and Feminist Philosophy*, ed. Catriona Mackenzie, Wendy Rogers, and Susan Dodds (New York: Oxford University Press, 2014), 79.

62. Exercise is one of the activities that Deborah K. Padgett, Benjamin F. Henwood, and Sam J. Tsemberis identify as requiring a person to have a stable home to participate in. Deborah K. Padgett, Benjamin F. Henwood, and Sam J. Tsemberis, *Housing First: Ending Homelessness, Transforming Systems, and Changing Lives* (Oxford: Oxford University Press, 2016), 173.

63. Gosselin, *Mental Patient*, 65–67.

Chapter 3: Inner Resources

1. Saks, *The Center Cannot Hold*, 322.
2. Steele and Berman, *The Day the Voices Stopped*, 173.
3. Steele and Berman, *The Day the Voices Stopped*, 137.
4. Steele and Berman, *The Day the Voices Stopped*, 177.
5. Steele and Berman, *The Day the Voices Stopped*, 181.
6. Susanne Schwager and Klaus Rothermund identify changing a difficult situation as assimilative coping and changing one's appraisal of a situation (which can be an aspect of changing oneself to adjust to a situation better) as accommodative coping. Susanne Schwager and Klaus Rothermund, "The Automatic Basis of Resilience: Adaptive Regulation of Affect and Cognition," in *The Resilience Handbook: Approaches to Stress and Trauma*, ed. Martha Kent, Mary C. Davis, and John W. Reich (New York: Routledge, 2014), 57–58.

7. Juli T. Eflin, "An Epistemological Base for the Problem Solving Model of Creativity," *Philosophica* 64, no. 2 (1999): 51–52; Linda Trinkaus Zagzebski, *Virtues of the Mind: An Inquiry into the Nature of Virtue and the Ethical Foundations of Knowledge* (Cambridge: Cambridge University Press, 1996), 106–116.

Some virtue ethicists propose that virtues are like skills in the ways that we acquire and exercise them. For discussion of this, see Julia Annas, *Intelligent Virtue* (Oxford: Oxford University Press, 2011); Julia Annas, "Virtue as a Skill," *International Journal of Philosophical Studies* 3, no. 2 (1995): 227–243; Matt Stichter, "Ethical Expertise: The Skill Model of Virtue," *Ethical Theory and Moral Practice* 10 (2007): 183–194; Matt Stichter, "Virtues as Skills in Virtue Epistemology," *Journal of Philosophical Research* 38 (2013): 333–348.

8. Charles C. Benight and Roman Cieslak, "Cognitive Factors and Resilience: How Self-Efficacy Contributes to Coping with Adversities," in *Resilience and Mental Health: Challenges Across the Lifespan*, ed. Steven M. Southwick, Brett T. Litz, Dennis Charney, and Matthew J. Friedman (Cambridge: Cambridge University Press, 2011), 47; Colleen Willoughby, Elizabeth G. Brown, Gillian A. King, Jacqueline Specht, and Linda K. Smith, "The Resilient Self—What Helps and What Hinders?," in *Resilience: Learning from People with Disabilities and the Turning Points in Their Lives*, ed. Gillian A. King, Elizabeth G. Brown, and Linda K. Smith (Westport, CT: Praeger, 2003), 101.

9. Diana Tietjens Meyers, *Being Yourself: Essays on Identity, Action, and Social Life* (Lanham, MD: Rowman & Littlefield, 2004), 31.

10. Marilyn Friedman, "Autonomy, Social Disruption, and Women," in *Relational Autonomy: Feminist Perspectives on Autonomy, Agency, and the Social Self*, ed. Catriona Mackenzie and Natalie Stoljar (Oxford: Oxford University Press, 2000), 40.

11. Inga-Britt Lindh, António Barbosa da Silva, Agneta Berg, and Elisabeth Severinsson, "Courage and Nursing Practice: A Theoretical Analysis," *Nursing Ethics* 17, no. 5 (2010): 561.

12. Robert Audi, "Epistemological Dimensions of Intellectual Virtue," *Acta Philosophica* 27, no. 2 (2018): 231–232.

13. Havi Carel, *Illness: The Cry of the Flesh*, 3rd edition (London: Routledge, 2019), 99–106; Ian James Kidd, "Can Illness Be Edifying?," *Inquiry* 55, no. 5 (2012): 499–500.

14. Lotz, "Vulnerability and Resilience," 50.

15. Emily McRae, "Equanimity and Intimacy: A Buddhist-Feminist Approach to the Elimination of Bias," *Sophia* 52 (2013): 451–453.

16. McRae, "Equanimity and Intimacy," 451; Neil Pembroke, "Compassionate Care by Clinicians: Insights from the Judeo-Christian and Buddhist Traditions," *Eubios Journal of Asian and International Bioethics* 25, no. 1 (January 2015): 22–23.

17. Pembroke, "Compassionate Care by Clinicians," 23; McRae, "Equanimity and Intimacy," 451.

18. Songyao Ren, "The Zhuangist Views on Emotions," *Asian Philosophy* 28, no. 1 (2018): 58.

19. Emily McRae, "Equanimity and the Moral Virtue of Open-Mindedness," *American Philosophical Quarterly* 53, no. 1 (January 2016): 98–99.

20. McRae, "Equanimity and the Moral Virtue of Open-Mindedness," 97–108.

21. Epictetus, *Enchiridion*, trans. George Long (Mineola, NY: Dover, 2004), 4 (aphorism 8).

22. Derk Pereboom, "Stoic Psychotherapy in Descartes and Spinoza," *Faith and Philosophy: Journal of the Society of Christian Philosophers* 11, no. 4 (1994): Article 4, doi: 10.5840/faithphil199411444, 593.

23. Lewis Ross, "The Virtue of Curiosity," *Episteme* 17, no. 1 (2020): 108–109.

24. Richard Phillips, "Curiosity: Care, Virtue and Pleasure in Uncovering the New," *Theory, Culture & Society* 32, no. 3 (2015): 149–161.

25. Elias Baumgarten, "Curiosity as a Moral Virtue," *International Journal of Applied Philosophy* 15, no. 2 (2001): 171–172.

26. Baumgarten, "Curiosity as a Moral Virtue," 173.

27. Aristotle, *Nicomachean Ethics*, trans. Robert C. Bartlett and Susan D. Collins (Chicago: University of Chicago Press, 2011), 56 (book 3, chapter 7).

28. Lear, *Radical Hope*, 109–113.

29. Giles Pearson, "Aristotle on the Role of Confidence in Courage," *Ancient Philosophy* 29 (2009): 136.

30. Steele and Berman, *The Day the Voices Stopped*, 204. Doug McConnell and Anke Snoek support Ken Steele's claim that change is difficult when a person is used to being sick and in treatment because their identity comes to be wrapped up in their illness and its treatment. In the context of addiction, a person's identity revolves around their addictive behavior; changing the behavior requires changing their identity, and this can be very hard to do. Doug McConnell and Anke Snoek, "The Importance of Self-Narration in Recovery from Addiction," *Philosophy, Psychiatry, & Psychology* 25, no. 3 (September 2018): E31–E44.

31. Steele and Berman, *The Day the Voices Stopped*, 204.

32. For discussion of perseverance in an epistemic context, see Heather Battaly, "Intellectual Perseverance," *Journal of Moral Philosophy* 14 (2017): 669–697.

33. Piper S. Meyer and Kim T. Mueser, "Resiliency in Individuals with Serious Mental Illness," in *Resilience and Mental Health: Challenges Across the Lifespan*, ed. Steven M. Southwick, Brett T. Litz, Dennis Charney, and Matthew J. Friedman (Cambridge: Cambridge University Press, 2011), 279.

34. Ariel Meirav, "The Nature of Hope," *Ratio* 22 (June 2009): 219; Michael Milona, "Discovering the Virtue of Hope," *European Journal of Philosophy* 28 (2020): 741, doi: 10.1111/ejop.12518.

35. Claudia Blöser, Jakob Huber, and Darrel Moellendorf, "Hope in Political Philosophy," *Philosophy Compass* 15, no. e12665 (2020): 2, https://doi.org/10.1111/phc3.12665.

36. Carl-Johan Palmqvist, "Faith and Hope in Situations of Epistemic Uncertainty," *Religious Studies* 55 (2019): 331.

37. Meirav, "The Nature of Hope," 219.

38. Hope is also compatible with a belief that the future will be bad. Michael Schrader and Michael Levine, "Hope: The Janus Faced Virtue (with Feathers)," *European Journal for Philosophy of Religion* 11, no. 3 (2019): 18–19.

39. Margaret Urban Walker, "Hope's Value," in *Moral Repair: Reconstructing Moral Relations after Wrongdoing* (Cambridge: Cambridge University Press, 2006), 48.

40. Luc Bovens, "The Value of Hope," *Philosophy and Phenomenological Research* 59, no. 3 (September 1999): 674.

41. Tamar Szabó Gendler, "Alief in Action (and Reaction)," *Mind & Language* 23, no. 5 (2008): 552–585. See also Miri Albahari, "Alief or Belief? A Contextual Approach to Belief Ascription," *Philosophical Studies* 167 (2014): 701–720.

42. Blöser, Huber, and Moellendorf, "Hope in Political Philosophy," 3–4.

43. Adam Kavlac, "The Virtue of Hope," *Ethical Theory and Moral Practice* 18 (2015): 343.

44. Milona, "Discovering the Virtue of Hope," 744.

45. Milona, "Discovering the Virtue of Hope," 747–749.

46. Joan Woolfrey describes hope as "infectious." Joan Woolfrey, "The Infectiousness of Hope," *Philosophy in the Contemporary World* 22, no. 2 (Fall 2015): 94–103.

47. Walker, "Hope's Value," 41.

48. Adrienne M. Martin, *How We Hope: A Moral Psychology* (Princeton, NJ: Princeton University Press, 2014), 25 and 61–69.

49. Martin, *How We Hope*, 65. See also Philip Pettit, "Hope and Its Place in Mind," *Annals of the American Academy* 592 (March 2004): 152–165, doi: 10.11.77/0002716203261798.

50. Blöser, Huber, and Moellendorf, "Hope in Political Philosophy," 4.

51. Jack M. C. Kwong, "What Is Hope?," *European Journal of Philosophy* 27 (2019): 246–248.

52. G. Scott Gravlee, "Aristotle on Hope," *Journal of the History of Philosophy* 38, no. 4 (October 2000): 461–477.

53. Julie Repper and Rachel Perkins, *Social Inclusion and Recovery: A Model for Mental Health Practice* (Edinburgh: Ballière Tindall, 2003), 48–50; Mike Slade, *Personal Recovery and Mental Illness: A Guide for Mental Health Professionals* (Cambridge: Cambridge University Press, 2009), 77.

54. Repper and Perkins, *Social Inclusion and Recovery*, 51–58.

Chapter 4: Social Support

1. Saks, *The Center Cannot Hold*, 263.
2. Saks, *The Center Cannot Hold*, 123.
3. Saks, *The Center Cannot Hold*, 167.
4. Saks, *The Center Cannot Hold*, 183.
5. Saks, *The Center Cannot Hold*, 271.
6. Saks, *The Center Cannot Hold*, 271.

7. Stephen A. Stansfeld, "Social Support and Social Cohesion," in *Social Determinants of Health*, 2nd edition, ed. Michael Marmot and Richard G. Wilkinson (Oxford: Oxford University Press, 2006), 158–160. See also Southwick and Charney, *Resilience*, 145–146.

8. Stansfeld, "Social Support and Social Cohesion," 150.

9. Denise Janicki-Deverts and Sheldon Cohen, "Social Ties and Resilience in Chronic Disease," in *Resilience and Mental Health: Challenges Across the Lifespan*, ed. Steven M. Southwick, Brett T. Litz, Dennis Charney, and Matthew J. Friedman (Cambridge: Cambridge University Press, 2011), 77–79; Stansfeld, "Social Support and Social Cohesion," 151–152.

10. Janicki-Deverts and Cohen, "Social Ties and Resilience in Chronic Disease," 78.

11. Janicki-Deverts and Cohen, "Social Ties and Resilience in Chronic Disease," 77–78; Stansfeld, "Social Support and Social Cohesion," 151–152.

12. Studies cited in Glicken, *Learning from Resilient People*, 102.

13. Vicki S. Helgeson and Lindsey Lopez, "Social Support and Growth Following Adversity," in *Handbook of Adult Resilience*, ed. John W. Reich, Alex J. Zautra, and John Stuart Hall (New York: Guilford Press, 2010), 310; Meera Padhy and Padiri Ruth Angiel, "Social Support and Emotion Regulation as Predictors of Well-Being," in *Emotion, Well-Being, and Resilience: Theoretical Perspectives and Practical Applications*, ed. Rabindra Kumar Pradhan and Updesh Kumar (Palm Bay, FL: Apple Academic Press, 2021), 62–63.

14. Barrett Emerick, "Empathy and a Life of Moral Endeavor," *Hypatia* 31, no. 2 (Winter 2016): 171–186; Peter Goldie, *The Emotions: A Philosophical Exploration* (Oxford: Clarendon Press, 2000), 178; Jean Harvey, "Moral Solidarity and Empathetic Understanding," *Journal of Social Philosophy* 38, no. 1 (Spring 2007): 22–37.

15. Brian Carr, "Pity and Compassion as Social Virtues," *Philosophy* 74 (1999): 411–429; Roger Crisp, "Compassion and Beyond," *Ethical Theory and Moral Practice* 11 (2008): 233–246.

16. Helgeson and Lopez, "Social Support and Growth Following Adversity," 314.

17. Helgeson and Lopez, "Social Support and Growth Following Adversity," 313.

18. Saks, *The Center Cannot Hold*, 148–162.

19. Saks, *The Center Cannot Hold*, 201.

20. Robert E. Goodin, *Protecting the Vulnerable: A Reanalysis of Our Social Responsibilities* (Chicago: University of Chicago Press, 1985). For a briefer summary of the arguments made in his book, see also Robert E. Goodin, "Vulnerabilities and Responsibilities: An Ethical Defense of the Welfare State," in *Necessary Goods: Our Responsibilities to Meet Others' Needs*, ed. Gillian Brock (Lanham, MD: Rowman & Littlefield, 1998), 73–94.

21. Goodin, *Protecting the Vulnerable*, 112.

22. Goodin, *Protecting the Vulnerable*, 112.

23. Goodin, *Protecting the Vulnerable*, 113.

24. Goodin, *Protecting the Vulnerable*, 114.

25. Goodin, *Protecting the Vulnerable*, 114.

26. Goodin, *Protecting the Vulnerable*, 115.
27. Goodin, *Protecting the Vulnerable*, 130.
28. Goodin, *Protecting the Vulnerable*, 118.
29. Goodin, *Protecting the Vulnerable*, 192.
30. Goodin, *Protecting the Vulnerable*, 192–193.
31. Goodin, *Protecting the Vulnerable*, 127.
32. Goodin, *Protecting the Vulnerable*, 128.
33. Goodin, *Protecting the Vulnerable*, 129.
34. Goodin, *Protecting the Vulnerable*, 130.
35. Gosselin, *Mental Patient*, 50.
36. Goodin, *Protecting the Vulnerable*, 132.
37. Goodin, *Protecting the Vulnerable*, 133.
38. Goodin, *Protecting the Vulnerable*, 151–153.
39. Sarah Clark Miller, *The Ethics of Need: Agency, Dignity, and Obligation* (New York: Routledge, 2012).
40. Miller, *The Ethics of Need*, 54–55.
41. Miller, *The Ethics of Need*, 57.
42. Miller, *The Ethics of Need*, 52–56.
43. Susan J. Brison, *Aftermath: Violence and the Remaking of a Self* (Princeton, NJ: Princeton University Press, 2002), 49–59.
44. Petra Gelhaus, "The Desired Moral Attitude of the Physician: (I) Empathy," *Medicine, Health Care and Philosophy* 15 (2012): 103–113; Jodi Halpern, *From Detached Concern to Empathy: Humanizing Medical Practice* (Oxford: Oxford University Press, 2001), 17.
45. Petra Gelhaus, "The Desired Moral Attitude of the Physician: (II) Compassion," *Medicine, Health Care and Philosophy* 15 (2012): 400.
46. Carr, "Pity and Compassion as Social Virtues," 411.
47. Halpern, "From Idealized Clinical Empathy to Empathic Communication in Medical Care."
48. Emerick, "Empathy and a Life of Moral Endeavor," 171–186; Goldie, *The Emotions*, 178; Harvey, "Moral Solidarity and Empathetic Understanding," 22–37; Meyers, *Being Yourself*, 115; Aaron Simmons, "In Defense of the Moral Significance of Empathy," *Ethical Theory and Moral Practice* 17 (2014): 97–111; Nancy Snow, "Empathy," *American Philosophical Quarterly* 37, no. 1 (2000): 65–78.
49. Carr, "Pity and Compassion as Social Virtues," 411–429; Crisp, "Compassion and Beyond," 233–246.
50. Miller, *The Ethics of Need*, 74–76.
51. Miller, *The Ethics of Need*, 78.
52. Miller, *The Ethics of Need*, 52.
53. Miller, *The Ethics of Need*, 61.
54. Miller, *The Ethics of Need*, 82.
55. Miller, *The Ethics of Need*, 53–54.

56. Miller, *The Ethics of Need*, 61–62.
57. Miller, *The Ethics of Need*, 62.
58. Miller, *The Ethics of Need*, 62–63.
59. Miller, *The Ethics of Need*, 64.
60. Miller, *The Ethics of Need*, 63.
61. Miller, *The Ethics of Need*, 74 and 83–86.
62. Immanuel Kant, *Grounding for the Metaphysics of Morals*, 3rd edition, trans. James W. Ellington (Indianapolis, IN: Hackett, 1993), 44–45.
63. Paul W. Taylor, *Respect for Nature: A Theory of Environmental Ethics*, 25th Anniversary Edition (Princeton, NJ: Princeton University Press, 1986), 61–75.
64. Robert Elliot, "Normative Ethics," in *A Companion to Environmental Philosophy*, ed. Dale Jamieson (Malden, MA: Blackwell, 2003), 180.
65. Miller, *The Ethics of Need*, 88–95.

Chapter 5: Resources for Meeting People's Needs

1. Steele and Berman, *The Day the Voices Stopped*, 57.
2. Alan Gewirth, *Human Rights: Essays on Justification and Applications* (Chicago: University of Chicago Press, 1982).

Gewirth's approach is similar to James Griffin's theory of human rights, in which he grounds human rights on "personhood," understanding personhood as having "normative agency." Griffin defines normative agency as "the agency involved in living a worthwhile life." James Griffin, *On Human Rights* (Oxford: Oxford University Press, 2008), 45.

As the agency involved in living a worthwhile life involves having the capacity to identify the good, normative agency can be understood as what I called autonomous agency in chapter 2. Rights protect the interests involved with autonomy and liberty, which are required for normative agency. Griffin, *On Human Rights*, 33–48.

3. Gewirth, *Human Rights*, 51–52.
4. Gewirth, *Human Rights*, 52.
5. Gewirth, *Human Rights*, 55.
6. Gewirth, *Human Rights*, 55–56.
7. Gewirth, *Human Rights*, 56.
8. Gewirth, *Human Rights*, 56.
9. United Nations, "International Covenant on Economic, Social and Cultural Rights," United Nations Human Rights Office of the High Commissioner, ratified 1966, accessed August 8, 2022, https://www.ohchr.org/sites/default/files/Documents/ProfessionalInterest/cescr.pdf.
10. United Nations, "International Covenant on Economic, Social and Cultural Rights."

11. Thomas W. Pogge, *World Poverty and Human Rights: Cosmopolitan Responsibilities and Reforms*, 2nd edition (Cambridge: Polity, 2008), 52 and 70–71.

12. Mikaela Heikkilä, Hisayo Katsui, and Maija Mustaniemi-Laakso, "Disability and Vulnerability: A Human Rights Reading of the Responsive State," *International Journal of Human Rights* 24, no. 8 (2020): 1185.

13. Henry Shue, *Basic Rights: Subsistence, Affluence, and U.S. Foreign Policy* (Princeton, NJ: Princeton University Press, 1980), 52–53. Using Shue's framework, the right to mental health can be understood as a security right that must be fulfilled in order for a person to have "physical security." Since the physical and mental are intertwined, physical security can only be attained with concurrent mental security. Mental health is needed for mental security.

For discussion of the three correlative duties Shue identifies, see Thomas Pogge, "Are We Violating the Human Rights of the World's Poor?," *Yale Human Rights and Development Journal* 14, no. 2 (2011): 5 (Article 1), accessed February 17, 2022, http://digitalcommons.law.yale.edu/yhrdlj/vol14/iss2/1.

14. Onora O'Neill, *Towards Justice and Virtue: A Constructive Account of Practical Reasoning* (Cambridge: Cambridge University Press, 1996), 128–136. See also Onora O'Neill, "Rights, Obligations, and Needs," in *Necessary Goods: Our Responsibilities to Meet Others' Needs*, ed. Gillian Brock (Lanham, MD: Rowman & Littlefield, 1998), 95–112.

15. Gewirth, *Human Rights*, 209.

16. Michael Green, "Institutional Responsibility for Moral Problems," in *Global Responsibilities: Who Must Deliver on Human Rights?*, ed. Andrew Kuper (New York: Routledge, 2005), 123.

17. Green, "Institutional Responsibility for Moral Problems," 124.

18. Elizabeth Ashford, "The Duties Imposed by the Human Right to Basic Necessities," in *Freedom from Poverty as a Human Right: Who Owes What to the Very Poor?*, ed. Thomas Pogge (Oxford: Oxford University Press, 2007), 197.

19. Some critics may be concerned that a rights approach is not a productive approach to take in discourse around mental health needs and obligations because it can create adversarial relationships, especially in the context of mental health professionals and their patients, and it can shape discourse around competing rights claims that are hard to adjudicate. I believe that a rights approach is an important dimension for thinking about resilience, however, because it gives people a basis for making claims (rights claims) based on their needs in a way that obligates others to fulfill their rights/meet their needs. Thus, a rights approach is empowering to vulnerable people. I agree that a rights approach can be adversarial, which can detract from productive conversations about meeting people's needs, but it need not be, particularly when it is used to understand the relationship between vulnerable individuals and the institutions that shape their lives.

A rights approach can clarify who has obligations and on what basis. In the present context, a rights approach shows that institutions have significant obligations in meeting the right to mental health that can be overlooked when we focus on individual duties like the duty to protect the vulnerable and the duty to care. While dominant deontological and consequentialist approaches to supporting vulnerable people do a good job identifying what individuals should do for vulnerable people, a human rights approach can better identify what institutions should do. An analysis of the social context of resilience would be incomplete without an analysis of institutional responsibilities related to resilience; a rights approach provides a way to ground institutional responsibilities for addressing vulnerability. Thus, while a rights approach might not be the most effective or meaningful way to frame relationships between service providers and clients, or mental health professionals and their patients, it is nonetheless an important way to understand the responsibilities that institutions and systems have toward those with mental illness.

20. Martha Albertson Fineman, "Equality, Autonomy, and the Vulnerable Subject in Law and Politics," in *Vulnerability: Reflections on a New Ethical Foundation for Law and Politics*, ed. Martha Albertson Fineman and Anna Grear (Farnham, England: Ashgate, 2013), 13–27; Fineman, "The Vulnerable Subject," 1–23; Martha Albertson Fineman, "The Vulnerable Subject and the Responsive State," *Emory Law Journal* 60 (2010): 251–275.

21. Turner, *Vulnerability and Human Rights*.

22. Fineman, "The Vulnerable Subject and the Responsive State," 265.

23. Fineman, "The Vulnerable Subject and the Responsive State," 269.

24. Fineman, "The Vulnerable Subject," 13–15; Fineman, "The Vulnerable Subject and the Responsive State," 270–271.

25. Fineman, "The Vulnerable Subject," 15.

26. Fineman, "The Vulnerable Subject," 16.

27. Fineman, "The Vulnerable Subject," 18.

28. Heikkilä, Katsui, and Mustaniemi-Laakso, "Disability and Vulnerability," 1189.

29. Fineman, "The Vulnerable Subject and the Responsive State," 272.

30. Fineman, "The Vulnerable Subject and the Responsive State," 272.

31. Fineman, "The Vulnerable Subject," 19.

32. Fineman, "The Vulnerable Subject," 19.

33. Monique Deveaux, "The Global Poor as Agents of Justice," *Journal of Moral Philosophy* 12 (2015): 125–150; Alejandra Mancilla, "The Human Right to Subsistence," *Philosophy Compass* 14 (2019): e12618, 1–10, accessed August 8, 2022, https://compass.onlinelibrary.wiley.com/doi/10.1111/phc3.12618.

34. Monique Deveaux makes this argument in the context of meeting the needs and fulfilling the human rights of the global poor. Deveaux, "The Global Poor as Agents of Justice."

35. Anastasia Philippa Scrutton, "Epistemic Injustice and Mental Illness," in *The Routledge Handbook of Epistemic Injustice*, ed. Ian James Kidd, Jose Medina, and Gaile Pohlhaus Jr. (London: Routledge, 2017), 347–355.

36. Şerife Tekin, "Patients as Experience-Based Experts in Psychiatry: Insights from the Natural Method," in *The Natural Method: Essays on Mind, Ethics, and Self in Honor of Owen Flanagan*, ed. Eddy Nahmias, Thomas W. Polger, and Wenqing Zhao (Cambridge, MA: MIT Press, 2020), 88.

37. Alejandra Mancilla identifies this goal as one of the goals of people who are poor, who act as agents on their own behalf to get their right to subsistence met. Mancilla, "The Human Right to Subsistence," 6.

Chapter 6: Resources for Social Justice

1. Marc Fleurbaey describes this kind of economic exploitation, when the poor are given options they cannot refuse because there are no better options. Marc Fleurbaey, "Poverty as a Form of Oppression," in *Freedom from Poverty as a Human Right: Who Owes What to the Very Poor?*, ed. Thomas Pogge (Oxford and New York: Oxford University Press, 2007), 144–145.

2. Steele and Berman, *The Day the Voices Stopped*, 40–50 and 105–106.

3. Steele and Berman, *The Day the Voices Stopped*, 91–97, 105–106, and 115.

4. There are limited programs that try to give people in need housing irrespective of social problems they are dealing with. The Housing First approach, which has been adopted on a small scale in various communities throughout the world, provides homeless people with housing before attending to other needs such as mental health treatment, substance use treatment, obtaining employment, or obtaining food security. "Housing First," National Alliance to End Homelessness, April 20, 2016, accessed April 1, 2022, https://endhomelessness.org/resource/housing-first/?msclkid=a2c7065db20011ec8efb938e6962f5e0; Padgett, Henwood, and Tsemberis, *Housing First*.

5. Steele lived during a time before the invention and use of cellphones.

6. There are pilot programs across the United States that give money with no strings attached to low-income people, and they have been successful at reducing poverty, improving housing, decreasing food insecurity, and enabling childcare. Kalena Thomhave, "Money for the People," *The Progressive* (June/July 2021): 41–44. Some of the pandemic relief money was directed toward this purpose as well. Attitudes since the pandemic have shifted as more Americans find giving money with no strings attached, especially to low-income people, to be acceptable and worthwhile. Donald R. Richards and Thomas L. Steiger, "Value Orientations and Support for Guaranteed Income," *Social Science Quarterly* 102 (2021): 2733–2751.

7. Steele and Berman, *The Day the Voices Stopped*, 151, 158–160, and 173–181.

8. Saks, *The Center Cannot Hold*, 148–162; Steele and Berman, *The Day the Voices Stopped*, 52–60 and 116.

9. Steele and Berman, *The Day the Voices Stopped*, 79–81.

10. Steele and Berman, *The Day the Voices Stopped*, 116–117.

11. Ruth S. Shim and Michael T. Compton, "The Social Determinants of Mental Health: Psychiatrists' Roles in Addressing Discrimination and Food Insecurity," *Focus* 18, no. 1 (Winter 2020): 25.

12. Jessica Allen, Reuben Balfour, Ruth Bell, and Michael Marmot, "Social Determinants of Mental Health," *International Review of Psychiatry* 26, no. 4 (August 2014): 392–407; Michael T. Compton and Ruth S. Shim, "Mental Illness Prevention and Mental Health Promotion: When, Who, and How," *Psychiatric Services* 71, no. 9 (September 2020): 981; Ellen Fink-Samnick, "The Social Determinants of Mental Health: Definitions, Distinctions, and Dimensions for Professional Case Management: Part 1," *Professional Case Management* 26, no. 3 (2021): 121; Matthew Fisher and Fran Baum, "The Social Determinants of Mental Health: Implications for Research and Health Promotion," *Australian and New Zealand Journal of Psychiatry* 44, no. 12 (December 2010): 1058; Emma Motrico, Jose A. Salinas-Perez, Maria Luisa Rodero-Cosano, and Sonia Conejo-Cerón, "Editors' Comments on the Special Issue 'Social Determinants of Mental Health,'" *International Journal of Environmental Research and Public Health* 18, no. 3957 (2021): 1, https://doi.org/10.3390/ijerph18083957; Ruth S. Shim and Michael T. Compton, "Addressing the Social Determinants of Mental Health: If Not Now, When? If Not Us, Who?," *Psychiatric Services* 69, no. 8 (August 2018): 844; Shim and Compton, "The Social Determinants of Mental Health," 25. See also Michael Marmot and Richard G. Wilkinson, *Social Determinants of Health*, 2nd edition (Oxford: Oxford University Press, 2006); and Kathryn Strother Ratcliff, *The Social Determinants of Health: Looking Upstream* (Cambridge: Polity Press, 2017).

13. Fisher and Baum, "The Social Determinants of Mental Health," 1057–1063. See also Margarita Alegria, Amanda NeMoyer, Irene Falgàs Bagué, Ye Wang, and Kiara Alvarez, "Social Determinants of Mental Health: Where We Are and Where We Need to Go," *Current Psychiatry Reports* 20, no. 95 (2018): 1, accessed February 23, 2022, https://doi.org/10.1007/s11920-018-0969-9; Lloyd I. Sederer, "The Social Determinants of Mental Health," *Psychiatric Services* 67, no. 2 (February 2016): 234–235.

14. Compton and Shim, "Mental Illness Prevention and Mental Health Promotion," 981.

15. Shim and Compton, "The Social Determinants of Mental Health," 26.

16. Shim and Compton, "Addressing the Social Determinants of Mental Health," 845.

17. Shim and Compton, "The Social Determinants of Mental Health," 25.

18. Shim and Compton, "Addressing the Social Determinants of Mental Health," 844.

19. Alegria, NeMoyer, Bagué, Wang, and Alvarez, "Social Determinants of Mental Health," 3; Fink-Samnick, "The Social Determinants of Mental Health," 130.

20. Iris Marion Young, *Responsibility for Justice* (Oxford: Oxford University Press, 2011), 38.

21. Young, *Responsibility for Justice*, 52.

22. Young, *Responsibility for Justice*, 45.

23. Young, *Responsibility for Justice*, 45.

24. Fleurbaey, "Poverty as a Form of Oppression," 144–145.

25. Young, *Responsibility for Justice*, 55.

26. Of course, sometimes harm comes from specific decisions made by, and specific actions implemented by, specific individuals carrying out their role responsibilities within institutions. Harmful decisions and actions can result from a corrupting influence the role has on the individuals carrying out the role, or from the role attracting corrupt individuals who are willing to enact unjust policies, perhaps for personal gain. In some cases, individuals within these roles may be culpable for causing harm through their bad choices and actions. In such cases, removing bad actors from these roles or changing the power structure of the roles can create the desired change of improving the institution's practices.

However, because of the way power and decision-making is often dispersed within an institution, it can sometimes be very difficult to identify specific agents who are culpable and therefore liable for their choices and actions. The dispersed responsibility that arises from the structure of many institutions makes holding specific individuals responsible very difficult, which is why structural responsibility often better accounts for the responsibilities that institutions have.

27. Young, *Responsibility for Justice*, 60.

28. Young focuses on the duties of structural justice that individuals have, while Christian Neuhäuser emphasizes that institutions have duties of structural justice as well. Christian Neuhäuser, "Structural Injustice and the Distribution of Forward-Looking Responsibility," *Midwest Studies in Philosophy* 38 (2014): 232–251.

29. Iris Marion Young identifies five types of oppression: exploitation, marginalization, powerlessness, cultural imperialism, and violence. All are relevant to people with mental illness, and being subject to any of these types of oppression can contribute to increased stress and poorer mental health. Iris M. Young, "Five Faces of Oppression," *Philosophical Forum* 19, no. 6 (1988): 270–290.

30. Erving Goffman, *Asylums: Essays on the Social Situation of Mental Patients and Other Inmates* (New York: Anchor Books, 1961), 6.

31. Young, *Responsibility for Justice*, 104–113.

32. Michael Doan describes the epistemic dimensions of political struggle, noting that epistemic justice is not only a matter of interpersonal justice between different epistemic participants, but also a matter of structural justice between

individuals and the institutions and systems with which they interact. Michael Doan, "Resisting Structural Epistemic Injustice," *Feminist Philosophy Quarterly* 4, no. 4 (2018): 1–23 (Article 5).

33. Fricker, *Epistemic Injustice*, 9–29.

34. Joseph Beatty, "Good Listening," *Educational Theory* 49, no. 3 (Summer 1999): 282.

35. Beatty, "Good Listening," 282.

36. Susan E. Notess, "Listening to People: Using Social Psychology to Spotlight an Overlooked Virtue," *Philosophy* 94, no. 370 (October 2019): 621–643.

37. Notess, "Listening to People," 641.

38. Notess, "Listening to People," 641.

39. Notess, "Listening to People," 621.

40. Notess, "Listening to People," 637 (italics original).

41. Beatty, "Good Listening," 285.

42. For example, listening in the context of dementia can involve trying to understand and foster the sense-making that the person with dementia is trying to achieve rather than trying to convince them of the "truth" of their situation. Matthews and Kennett, "Respecting Agency in Dementia Care."

43. Nancy Nyquist Potter, "Voice, Silencing, and Listening Well: Socially Located Patients, Oppressive Structures, and an Invitation to Shift the Epistemic Terrain," in *The Bloomsbury Companion to Philosophy of Psychiatry*, ed. Şerife Tekin and Robyn Bluhm (London: Bloomsbury Academic, 2019), 305–324. See also Paul Crichton, Havi Carel, and Ian James Kidd, "Epistemic Injustice in Psychiatry," *British Journal of Psychiatry Bulletin* 41 (2017): 65–70.

44. Beatty, "Good Listening," 286.

45. Beatty, "Good Listening," 286.

46. Beatty, "Good Listening," 287.

47. Beatty, "Good Listening," 289. For more on understanding empathy as imaginatively reconstructing someone else's experience in order to understand their situation from their own point of view, see Emerick, "Empathy and a Life of Moral Endeavor," 171–186; Goldie, *The Emotions*, 178; Harvey, "Moral Solidarity and Empathetic Understanding," 22–37; Meyers, *Being Yourself*, 115; Simmons, "In Defense of the Moral Significance of Empathy," 97–111; Snow, "Empathy," 65–78.

48. Notess, "Listening to People," 629.

49. Notess, "Listening to People," 638.

50. Notess, "Listening to People," 639.

51. Lear, *Radical Hope*, 80.

52. Nancy Nyquist Potter, *The Virtue of Defiance and Psychiatric Engagement* (Oxford: Oxford University Press, 2016), 143.

53. Potter, *The Virtue of Defiance and Psychiatric Engagement*, 143.

54. Expressions should not be dismissed ("She's just bitter") as a way of marginalizing the concern of the person who is expressing their concern; their

concern, and the way it is expressed, must be taken seriously for it to be taken up appropriately. Sue Campbell, "Being Dismissed: The Politics of Emotional Expression," *Hypatia* 9, no. 3 (Summer 1994): 46–65.

Chapter 7: Opportunities for Meaning

1. Saks, *The Center Cannot Hold*, 247.
2. Saks, *The Center Cannot Hold*, 123 (italics original).
3. Saks, *The Center Cannot Hold*, 86–87.
4. Steele and Berman, *The Day the Voices Stopped*, 103.
5. Steele and Berman, *The Day the Voices Stopped*, 159–160.
6. Steele and Berman, *The Day the Voices Stopped*, 179.
7. Saks, *The Center Cannot Hold*, 104.
8. Saks, *The Center Cannot Hold*, 213.
9. Steele and Berman, *The Day the Voices Stopped*, 195.
10. Steele and Berman, *The Day the Voices Stopped*, 208–209.
11. Steele and Berman, *The Day the Voices Stopped*, 219–220.
12. Steele and Berman, *The Day the Voices Stopped*, 223.
13. Steele and Berman, *The Day the Voices Stopped*, 227–232.
14. Steele and Berman, *The Day the Voices Stopped*, 234.
15. Steele and Berman, *The Day the Voices Stopped*, 236.
16. Larry Davidson, "Considering Recovery as a Process: Or, Life Is Not an Outcome," in *Recovery of People with Mental Illness: Philosophical and Related Perspectives*, ed. Abraham Rudnick (Oxford: Oxford University Press, 2012), 252–263.
17. Rob Whitley and Robert Drake identify five dimensions of recovery that I discuss here: clinical, existential, functional, physical, and social dimensions of recovery. Rob Whitley and Robert E. Drake, "Recovery: A Dimensional Approach," *Psychiatric Services* 61, no. 12 (December 2010): 1248–1250.
18. Recovery is usually understood in terms of two broad categories: clinical and personal recovery. Here I am also considering other dimensions of recovery that are tied to these, using Whitley and Drake's approach (see previous note). For discussion of the difference between clinical and personal recovery, see Meyer and Mueser, "Resiliency in Individuals with Serious Mental Illness," 276–278; Slade, *Personal Recovery and Mental Illness*, 35–43. See also various discussions in Abraham Rudnick, ed., *Recovery of People with Mental Illness: Philosophical and Related Perspectives* (Oxford: Oxford University Press, 2012).
19. William A. Anthony, "Recovery from Mental Illness: The Guiding Vision of the Mental Health Service System in the 1990s," *Psychosocial Rehabilitation Journal* 16, no. 4 (April 1993): 20.
20. Patricia E. Deegan, "Recovery and Empowerment for People with Psychiatric Disabilities," *Social Work in Health Care* 25, no. 3 (1997): 20–21. See also

Patricia E. Deegan, "Recovery: The Lived Experience of Rehabilitation," *Psychosocial Rehabilitation Journal* 11, no. 4 (April 1988): 11–19.

21. Nora Jacobson and Dianne Greenley, "What Is Recovery? A Conceptual Model and Explication," *Psychiatric Services* 52, no. 4 (April 2001): 482–483; Whitley and Drake, "Recovery," 1248.

22. Jacobson and Greenley, "What Is Recovery?," 483; Whitley and Drake, "Recovery," 1248.

23. Viktor Frankl, *Man's Search for Meaning* (New York: Washington Square Press, 1984), 126.

24. Brian D. Ostafin and Travis Proulx, "Meaning in Life and Resilience to Stressors," *Anxiety, Stress, & Coping* 33, no. 6 (2020): 603–622.

25. Allison S. Troy and Iris B. Mauss, "Resilience in the Face of Stress: Emotion Regulation as a Protective Factor," in *Resilience and Mental Health: Challenges Across the Lifespan*, ed. Steven M. Southwick, Brett T. Litz, Dennis Charney, and Matthew J. Friedman (Cambridge: Cambridge University Press, 2011), 35.

26. Frankl, *Man's Search for Meaning*, 130–131.

27. Frankl, *Man's Search for Meaning*, 131.

28. Frankl, *Man's Search for Meaning*, 121 (italics original).

29. Gina Q. Boullion, Jeffrey M. Pavlacic, Stefan E. Schulenberg, Erin M. Buchanan, and Michael F. Steger, "Meaning, Social Support, and Resilience as Predictors of Posttraumatic Growth: A Study of the Louisiana Flooding of August 2016," *American Journal of Orthopsychiatry* 90, no. 5 (2020): 578–585; Marcela C. Weber, Jeffrey M. Pavlacic, Emily A. Gawlik, Stefan E. Schulenberg, and Erin M. Buchanan, "Modeling Resilience, Meaning in Life, Posttraumatic Growth, and Disaster Preparedness with Two Samples of Tornado Survivors," *Traumatology* 26, no. 3 (2020): 266–277.

30. Meyer and Mueser, "Resiliency in Individuals with Serious Mental Illness," 283.

31. Meyer and Mueser, "Resiliency in Individuals with Serious Mental Illness," 283–284.

32. Adeeba Hakkim and Amrita Deb, "Resilience through Meaning-Making: Case Studies of Childhood Adversity," *Psychological Studies* 66, no. 4 (October–December 2021): 423.

33. Hakkim and Deb, "Resilience through Meaning-Making," 423.

34. Meyer and Mueser, "Resiliency in Individuals with Serious Mental Illness," 284.

35. Gillian A. King, Tamzin Cathers, Elizabeth G. Brown, and Elizabeth MacKinnon, "Turning Points: Emotionally Compelling Life Experiences," in *Resilience: Learning from People with Disabilities and the Turning Points in Their Lives*, ed. Gillian A. King, Elizabeth G. Brown, and Linda K. Smith (Westport, CT: Praeger, 2003), 52–65.

36. For example, see her descriptions of her friendships with Kenny and Margie; Dinah, Patrick, and Sam; and Steve. Saks, *The Center Cannot Hold*, 44–45, 95–96, and 194–196.

37. For example, see his interactions with Nurse McCarthy, whose support led him to apply for—and obtain—a job, and his interactions with Rob, who helped him get back on his feet after being hospitalized. Steele and Berman, *The Day the Voices Stopped*, 98–102 and 146.

38. Willoughby, Brown, King, Specht, and Smith, "The Resilient Self—What Helps and What Hinders?," 94–110.

39. Dean Cocking and Jeanette Kennett explain how we develop our character and identity, as well as what is important to us and our conception of the good, based in part on how we relate to the people we are close to in our lives. Dean Cocking and Jeanette Kennett, "Friendship and the Self," *Ethics* 108, no. 3 (April 1998): 502–527.

40. Gosselin, *Humanizing Mental Illness*, 106–145.

41. Steele and Berman, *The Day the Voices Stopped*, 227.

42. Saks, *The Center Cannot Hold*, 336.

43. Saks, *The Center Cannot Hold*, 336.

44. Crystal L. Park and Jeanne M. Slattery, "Resilience Interventions with a Focus on Meaning and Values," in *The Resilience Handbook: Approaches to Stress and Trauma*, ed. Martha Kent, Mary C. Davis, and John W. Reich (New York: Routledge, 2014), 272.

45. Park and Slattery, "Resilience Interventions with a Focus on Meaning and Values," 272.

46. Park and Slattery, "Resilience Interventions with a Focus on Meaning and Values," 272.

47. Park and Slattery, "Resilience Interventions with a Focus on Meaning and Values," 272.

48. Park and Slattery, "Resilience Interventions with a Focus on Meaning and Values," 276.

49. Troy and Mauss, "Resilience in the Face of Stress," 37.

50. Troy and Mauss, "Resilience in the Face of Stress," 32.

51. Schwager and Rothermund, "The Automatic Basis of Resilience," 59.

52. Schwager and Rothermund, "The Automatic Basis of Resilience," 59.

53. Arthur W. Frank, *The Wounded Storyteller: Body, Illness, and Ethics* (Chicago: University of Chicago Press, 1995).

54. Hermione Thornhill, Linda Clare, and Rufus May, "Escape, Enlightenment and Endurance: Narratives of Recovery from Psychosis," *Anthropology & Medicine* 11, no. 2 (August 2004): 181–199.

55. Bruce MZ Cohen, *Mental Health User Narratives: New Perspectives on Illness and Recovery* (New York: Palgrave Macmillan, 2008), 150–153.

56. Gosselin, *Mental Patient*, 180–182.

57. Mohammed Abouelleil Rashed, *Madness and the Demand for Recognition: A Philosophical Inquiry into Identity and Mental Health Activism* (Oxford: Oxford University Press, 2019), 190–194. See also discussion in Gosselin, *Mental Patient*, 184–186.

58. Şerife Tekin, "Self-Concept through the Diagnostic Looking Glass: Narratives and Mental Disorder," *Philosophical Psychology* 24, no. 3 (June 2011): 357–380.

59. Tekin, "Self-Insight in the Time of Mood Disorders," 139–155.

60. Şerife Tekin, "The Missing Self in Scientific Psychiatry," *Synthese* 196 (2019): 2197–2215.

61. Tekin, "Self-Concept through the Diagnostic Looking Glass," 363–364.

62. James A. Montmarquet, *Epistemic Virtue and Doxastic Responsibility* (Lanham, MD: Rowman & Littlefield, 1993), 21.

63. Nicholas Manco and Sherry Hamby, "A Meta-Analytic Review of Interventions That Promote Meaning in Life," *American Journal of Health Promotion* 35, no. 6 (2021): 866–873.

64. Somayeh Moghbel Esfahani and Sayed Abbas Haghayegh, "The Effectiveness of Acceptance and Commitment Therapy on Resilience, Meaning in Life, and Family Function in Family Caregivers of Patients with Schizophrenia," *Quarterly of Horizon of Medical Sciences* 25, no. 4 (Autumn 2019): 298–311.

65. Park and Slattery, "Resilience Interventions with a Focus on Meaning and Values," 275.

66. Manco and Hamby, "A Meta-Analytic Review of Interventions That Promote Meaning in Life," 866–873.

67. Park and Slattery, "Resilience Interventions with a Focus on Meaning and Values," 273 and 278.

68. Robin Attfield notes that since work enables creativity and growth, the lack of opportunity for meaningful work is a harm as it inhibits personal development. Robin Attfield, "Work and the Human Essence," *Journal of Applied Philosophy* 1, no. 1 (1984): 147–148.

69. Larry Davidson and John S. Strauss, "Sense of Self in Recovery from Severe Mental Illness," in *Psychological and Social Aspects of Psychiatric Disability*, ed. LeRoy Spaniol, Cheryl Gagne, and Martin Koehler (Boston: Center for Psychiatric Rehabilitation [Boston University], 1997), 33.

70. Margaret Swarbrick, "A Wellness Approach to Mental Health Recovery," in *Recovery of People with Mental Illness: Philosophical and Related Perspectives*, ed. Abraham Rudnick (Oxford: Oxford University Press, 2012), 30–38.

71. Robert Pepper-Smith, William R. Harvey, and M. Silberfield, "Competency and Practical Judgment," *Theoretical Medicine* 17 (1996): 135–150; A. M. Guy Widdershoven, Andrea Ruissen, Anton J. L. M. van Balkom, and Gerben

Meynen, "Competence in Chronic Mental Illness: The Relevance of Practical Wisdom," *Journal of Medical Ethics* 43 (2017): 374–378.

72. Beth Angell, Andrea Cooke, and Kelly Kovac, "First-Person Accounts of Stigma," in *On the Stigma of Mental Illness: Practical Strategies for Research and Social Change*, ed. Patrick W. Corrigan (Washington, DC: American Psychological Association, 2005), 78–80.

73. Attfield, "Work and the Human Essence." See also discussions in James Rocha, "Autonomy within Subservient Careers," *Ethical Theory and Moral Practice* 14 (2011): 313–328; and Beate Roessler, "Meaningful Work: Arguments from Autonomy," *Journal of Political Philosophy* 20, no. 1 (2012): 71–93.

74. William Patrick Sullivan, "A Long and Winding Road: The Process of Recovery from Severe Mental Illness," in *Psychological and Social Aspects of Psychiatric Disability*, ed. LeRoy Spaniol, Cheryl Gagne, and Martin Koehler (Boston: Center for Psychiatric Rehabilitation [Boston University], 1997), 18–19.

75. Stephen P. Hinshaw, *The Mark of Shame: Stigma of Mental Illness and an Agenda for Change* (Oxford: Oxford University Press, 2007), 124.

76. Mihaly Csikszentmihalyi, *Flow: The Psychology of Optimal Experience* (New York: Harper Perennial, 1990).

77. Steve Matthews, Robyn Dwyer, and Anke Snoek explain how stigma and the fear of stigmatization lead to social isolation as well as exacerbation of mental illness symptoms in the context of addiction. Matthews, Dwyer, and Snoek, "Stigma and Self-Stigma in Addiction," 275–286.

78. Repper and Perkins, *Social Inclusion and Recovery*, 34.

79. Davidson and Strauss, "Sense of Self in Recovery from Severe Mental Illness," 25–39; Joan F. Houghton, "Maintaining Mental Health in a Turbulent World," in *Psychological and Social Aspects of Psychiatric Disability*, ed. LeRoy Spaniol, Cheryl Gagne, and Martin Koehler (Boston: Center for Psychiatric Rehabilitation [Boston University], 1997), 90.

80. Jeffrey Moriarty, "Rawls, Self-Respect, and the Opportunity for Meaningful Work," *Social Theory and Practice* 35, no. 3 (July 2009): 441–459.

81. Davidson and Strauss, "Sense of Self in Recovery from Severe Mental Illness," 25–39.

82. Moriarty, "Rawls, Self-Respect, and the Opportunity for Meaningful Work," 442.

83. Attfield, "Work and the Human Essence," 144–145; Moriarty, "Rawls, Self-Respect, and the Opportunity for Meaningful Work," 451.

84. Moriarty, "Rawls, Self-Respect, and the Opportunity for Meaningful Work," 442.

85. Hinshaw, *The Mark of Shame*, 124.

Bibliography

Albahari, Miri. "Alief or Belief? A Contextual Approach to Belief Ascription." *Philosophical Studies* 167 (2014): 701–720.

Alegria, Margarita, Amanda NeMoyer, Irene Falgàs Bagué, Ye Wang, and Kiara Alvarez. "Social Determinants of Mental Health: Where We Are and Where We Need to Go." *Current Psychiatry Reports* 20, no. 95 (2018): 1–13. Accessed February 23, 2022. https://doi.org/10.1007/s11920-018-0969-9.

Allen, Jessica, Reuben Balfour, Ruth Bell, and Michael Marmot. "Social Determinants of Mental Health." *International Review of Psychiatry* 26, no. 4 (August 2014): 392–407.

Anderson, Pamela Sue, Sabina Lovibond, and A. W. Moore. "Towards a New Philosophical Imaginary." *Angelaki: Journal of the Theoretical Humanities* 25, no. 1–2 (2020): 8–22.

Angell, Beth, Andrea Cooke, and Kelly Kovac. "First-Person Accounts of Stigma." In *On the Stigma of Mental Illness: Practical Strategies for Research and Social Change*, edited by Patrick W. Corrigan, 69–98. Washington, DC: American Psychological Association, 2005.

Annas, Julia. *Intelligent Virtue*. Oxford: Oxford University Press, 2011.

Annas, Julia. "Virtue as a Skill." *International Journal of Philosophical Studies* 3, no. 2 (1995): 227–243.

Anthony, William A. "Recovery from Mental Illness: The Guiding Vision of the Mental Health Service System in the 1990s." *Psychosocial Rehabilitation Journal* 16, no. 4 (April 1993): 11–23.

Aristotle. *Nicomachean Ethics*. Translated by Robert C. Bartlett and Susan D. Collins. Chicago: University of Chicago Press, 2011.

Ashford, Elizabeth. "The Duties Imposed by the Human Right to Basic Necessities." In *Freedom from Poverty as a Human Right: Who Owes What to the Very Poor?*, edited by Thomas Pogge, 183–218. Oxford: Oxford University Press, 2007.

Attfield, Robin. "Work and the Human Essence." *Journal of Applied Philosophy* 1, no. 1 (1984): 141–150.

Aubrecht, Katie. "The New Vocabulary of Resilience and the Governance of University Student Life." *Studies in Social Justice* 6, no. 1 (2012): 67–83.
Audi, Robert. "Epistemological Dimensions of Intellectual Virtue." *Acta Philosophica* 27, no. 2 (2018): 221–236.
Baiasu, Roxana. "The Openness of Vulnerability and Resilience." *Angelaki: Journal of the Theoretical Humanities* 25, no. 1–2 (2020): 254–264.
Battaly, Heather. "Intellectual Perseverance." *Journal of Moral Philosophy* 14 (2017): 669–697.
Baumgarten, Elias. "Curiosity as a Moral Virtue." *International Journal of Applied Philosophy* 15, no. 2 (2001): 169–184.
Beatty, Joseph. "Good Listening." *Educational Theory* 49, no. 3 (Summer 1999): 281–298.
Benight, Charles C., and Roman Cieslak. "Cognitive Factors and Resilience: How Self-Efficacy Contributes to Coping with Adversities." In *Resilience and Mental Health: Challenges Across the Lifespan*, edited by Steven M. Southwick, Brett T. Litz, Dennis Charney, and Matthew J. Friedman, 45–55. Cambridge: Cambridge University Press, 2011.
Bentall, Richard P. *Madness Explained: Psychosis and Human Nature*. New York: Penguin, 2003.
Blöser, Claudia, Jakob Huber, and Darrel Moellendorf. "Hope in Political Philosophy." *Philosophy Compass* 15, no. e12665 (2020): 1–9. https://doi.org/10.1111/phc3.12665.
Boullion, Gina Q., Jeffrey M. Pavlacic, Stefan E. Schulenberg, Erin M. Buchanan, and Michael F. Steger. "Meaning, Social Support, and Resilience as Predictors of Posttraumatic Growth: A Study of the Louisiana Flooding of August 2016." *American Journal of Orthopsychiatry* 90, no. 5 (2020): 578–585.
Bovens, Luc. "The Value of Hope." *Philosophy and Phenomenological Research* 59, no. 3 (September 1999): 667–681.
Boysen, Guy A., Erika L. Axtell, Abigail G. Kishimoto, and Breanna L. Sampo. "Generalized Perceptions of People with Mental Illness as Exploitable." *Evolutionary Behavioral Sciences* (2021). http://dx.doi.org/10.1037/ebs0000267.
Boysen, Guy A., and Raina A. Isaacs. "Perceptions of People with Mental Illness as Sexually Exploitable." *Evolutionary Behavioral Sciences* 16, no. 1 (2022): 38–52.
Brison, Susan J. *Aftermath: Violence and the Remaking of a Self*. Princeton, NJ: Princeton University Press, 2002.
Butler, Judith. "Rethinking Vulnerability and Resistance." In *Vulnerability in Resistance*, edited by Judith Butler, Zeynep Gambetti, and Leticia Sabsay, 12–27. Durham, NC: Duke University Press, 2016.
Campbell, Sue. "Being Dismissed: The Politics of Emotional Expression." *Hypatia* 9, no. 3 (Summer 1994): 46–65.
Carel, Havi. *Illness: The Cry of the Flesh*, 3rd edition. London: Routledge, 2019.

Carr, Brian. "Pity and Compassion as Social Virtues." *Philosophy* 74 (1999): 411–429.
Cocking, Dean, and Jeanette Kennett. "Friendship and the Self." *Ethics* 108, no. 3 (April 1998): 502–527.
Cohen, Bruce MZ. *Mental Health User Narratives: New Perspectives on Illness and Recovery*. New York: Palgrave Macmillan, 2008.
Compton, Michael T., and Ruth S. Shim. "Mental Illness Prevention and Mental Health Promotion: When, Who, and How." *Psychiatric Services* 71, no. 9 (September 2020): 981–983.
Corrigan, Patrick W., and Petra Kleinlein. "The Impact of Mental Illness Stigma." In *On the Stigma of Mental Illness: Practical Strategies for Research and Social Change*, edited by Patrick W. Corrigan, 11–44. Washington, DC: American Psychological Association, 2005.
Crichton, Paul, Havi Carel, and Ian James Kidd. "Epistemic Injustice in Psychiatry." *British Journal of Psychiatry Bulletin* 41 (2017): 65–70.
Crisp, Roger. "Compassion and Beyond." *Ethical Theory and Moral Practice* 11 (2008): 233–246.
Csikszentmihalyi, Mihaly. *Flow: The Psychology of Optimal Experience*. New York: Harper Perennial, 1990.
Davidson, Larry. "Considering Recovery as a Process: Or, Life Is Not an Outcome." In *Recovery of People with Mental Illness: Philosophical and Related Perspectives*, edited by Abraham Rudnick, 252–263. Oxford: Oxford University Press, 2012.
Davidson, Larry, and John S. Strauss. "Sense of Self in Recovery from Severe Mental Illness." In *Psychological and Social Aspects of Psychiatric Disability*, edited by LeRoy Spaniol, Cheryl Gagne, and Martin Koehler, 25–39. Boston: Center for Psychiatric Rehabilitation (Boston University), 1997.
Deegan, Patricia E. "Recovery and Empowerment for People with Psychiatric Disabilities." *Social Work in Health Care* 25, no. 3 (1997): 11–24.
Deegan, Patricia E. "Recovery: The Lived Experience of Rehabilitation." *Psychosocial Rehabilitation Journal* 11, no. 4 (April 1988): 11–19.
Deveaux, Monique. "The Global Poor as Agents of Justice." *Journal of Moral Philosophy* 12 (2015): 125–150.
Doan, Michael. "Resisting Structural Epistemic Injustice." *Feminist Philosophy Quarterly* 4, no. 4 (2018): 1–23 (Article 5).
Dodds, Susan. "Dependence, Care, and Vulnerability." In *Vulnerability: New Essays in Ethics and Feminist Philosophy*, edited by Catriona Mackenzie, Wendy Rogers, and Susan Dodds, 181–203. New York: Oxford University Press, 2014.
Dodson, Lisa. *The Moral Underground: How Ordinary Americans Subvert an Unfair Economy*. New York: New Press, 2011.
Eflin, Juli T. "An Epistemological Base for the Problem Solving Model of Creativity." *Philosophica* 64, no. 2 (1999): 49–63.

Elliot, Robert. "Normative Ethics." In *A Companion to Environmental Philosophy*, edited by Dale Jamieson, 177–191. Malden, MA: Blackwell, 2003.

Emerick, Barrett. "Empathy and a Life of Moral Endeavor." *Hypatia* 31, no. 2 (Winter 2016): 171–186.

Epictetus. *Enchiridion*. Translated by George Long. Mineola, NY: Dover, 2004.

Esfahani, Somayeh Moghbel, and Sayed Abbas Haghayegh. "The Effectiveness of Acceptance and Commitment Therapy on Resilience, Meaning in Life, and Family Function in Family Caregivers of Patients with Schizophrenia." *Quarterly of Horizon of Medical Sciences* 25, no. 4 (Autumn 2019): 298–311.

Fineman, Martha Albertson. "Equality, Autonomy, and the Vulnerable Subject in Law and Politics." In *Vulnerability: Reflections on a New Ethical Foundation for Law and Politics*, edited by Martha Albertson Fineman and Anna Grear, 13–27. Farnham, England: Ashgate, 2013.

Fineman, Martha Albertson. "The Vulnerable Subject: Anchoring Equality in the Human Condition." *Yale Journal of Law and Feminism* 20, no. 1 (2008): 1–23.

Fineman, Martha Albertson. "The Vulnerable Subject and the Responsive State." *Emory Law Journal* 60 (2010): 251–275.

Fink-Samnick, Ellen. "The Social Determinants of Mental Health: Definitions, Distinctions, and Dimensions for Professional Case Management: Part 1." *Professional Case Management* 26, no. 3 (2021): 121–137.

Fiorillo, Andrea, and Norman Sartorius. "Mortality Gap and Physical Comorbidity of People with Severe Mental Disorders: The Public Health Scandal." *Annals of General Psychiatry* 20, Article 52 (2021). Accessed October 4, 2023. https://annals-general-psychiatry.biomedcentral.com/articles/10.1186/s12991-021-00374-y.

Fisher, Matthew, and Fran Baum. "The Social Determinants of Mental Health: Implications for Research and Health Promotion." *Australian and New Zealand Journal of Psychiatry* 44, no. 12 (December 2010): 1057–1063.

Fleurbaey, Marc. "Poverty as a Form of Oppression." In *Freedom from Poverty as a Human Right: Who Owes What to the Very Poor?*, edited by Thomas Pogge, 133–154. Oxford: Oxford University Press, 2007.

Frank, Arthur W. *The Wounded Storyteller: Body, Illness, and Ethics*. Chicago: University of Chicago Press, 1995.

Frankl, Viktor. *Man's Search for Meaning*. New York: Washington Square Press, 1984.

Fricker, Miranda. *Epistemic Injustice: Power and the Ethics of Knowing*. Oxford: Oxford University Press, 2007.

Friedman, Marilyn. "Autonomy, Social Disruption, and Women." In *Relational Autonomy: Feminist Perspectives on Autonomy, Agency, and the Social Self*, edited by Catriona Mackenzie and Natalie Stoljar, 35–51. Oxford: Oxford University Press, 2000.

Gelhaus, Petra. "The Desired Moral Attitude of the Physician: (I) Empathy." *Medicine, Health Care and Philosophy* 15 (2012): 103–113.

Gelhaus, Petra. "The Desired Moral Attitude of the Physician: (II) Compassion." *Medicine, Health Care and Philosophy* 15 (2012): 397–410.
Gendler, Tamar Szabó. "Alief in Action (and Reaction)." *Mind & Language* 23, no. 5 (2008): 552–585.
Gewirth, Alan. *Human Rights: Essays on Justification and Applications*. Chicago: University of Chicago Press, 1982.
Gilson, Erinn C. *The Ethics of Vulnerability: A Feminist Analysis of Social Life and Practice*. New York: Routledge, 2014.
Glicken, Morley D. *Learning from Resilient People: Lessons We Can Apply to Counseling and Psychotherapy*. Thousand Oaks, CA: Sage, 2006.
Goffman, Erving. *Asylums: Essays on the Social Situation of Mental Patients and Other Inmates*. New York: Anchor Books, 1961.
Goldie, Peter. *The Emotions: A Philosophical Exploration*. Oxford: Clarendon Press, 2000.
Goodin, Robert E. *Protecting the Vulnerable: A Reanalysis of Our Social Responsibilities*. Chicago: University of Chicago Press, 1985.
Goodin, Robert E. "Vulnerabilities and Responsibilities: An Ethical Defense of the Welfare State." In *Necessary Goods: Our Responsibilities to Meet Others' Needs*, edited by Gillian Brock, 73–94. Lanham, MD: Rowman & Littlefield, 1998.
Gosselin, Abigail. *Humanizing Mental Illness: Enhancing Agency through Social Interaction*. Montreal: McGill-Queen's University Press, 2021.
Gosselin, Abigail. *Mental Patient: Psychiatric Ethics from a Patient's Perspective*. Cambridge, MA: MIT Press, 2022.
Gosselin, Abigail. "'A Useful Resource': Work Justice for People with Mental Illness." In *Peaceful Approaches for a More Peaceful World*, edited by Sanjay Lal, 239–269. Leiden: Brill, 2022.
Gravlee, G. Scott. "Aristotle on Hope." *Journal of the History of Philosophy* 38, no. 4 (October 2000): 461–477.
Green, Michael. "Institutional Responsibility for Moral Problems." In *Global Responsibilities: Who Must Deliver on Human Rights?*, edited by Andrew Kuper, 117–133. New York: Routledge, 2005.
Griffin, James. *On Human Rights*. Oxford: Oxford University Press, 2008.
Hakkim, Adeeba, and Amrita Deb. "Resilience through Meaning-Making: Case Studies of Childhood Adversity." *Psychological Studies* 66, no. 4 (October–December 2021): 422–433.
Halpern, Jodi. *From Detached Concern to Empathy: Humanizing Medical Practice*. Oxford: Oxford University Press, 2001.
Halpern, Jodi. "From Idealized Clinical Empathy to Empathic Communication in Medical Care." *Medicine, Health Care and Philosophy* 17 (2014): 301–311.
Harper, David, and Ewen Speed. "Uncovering Recovery: The Resistible Rise of Recovery and Resilience." *Studies in Social Justice* 6, no. 1 (2012): 9–25.

Harvey, Jean. "Moral Solidarity and Empathetic Understanding." *Journal of Social Philosophy* 38, no. 1 (Spring 2007): 22–37.

Heikkilä, Mikaela, Hisayo Katsui, and Maija Mustaniemi-Laakso. "Disability and Vulnerability: A Human Rights Reading of the Responsive State." *International Journal of Human Rights* 24, no. 8 (2020): 1180–1200.

Helgeson, Vicki S., and Lindsey Lopez. "Social Support and Growth Following Adversity." In *Handbook of Adult Resilience*, edited by John W. Reich, Alex J. Zautra, and John Stuart Hall, 309–330. New York: Guilford Press, 2010.

Hinshaw, Stephen P. *The Mark of Shame: Stigma of Mental Illness and an Agenda for Change*. Oxford: Oxford University Press, 2007.

"Homelessness and Housing." Substance Abuse and Mental Health Services Administration. Accessed August 8, 2022. https://www.samhsa.gov/homelessness-housing.

Houghton, Joan F. "Maintaining Mental Health in a Turbulent World." In *Psychological and Social Aspects of Psychiatric Disability*, edited by LeRoy Spaniol, Cheryl Gagne, and Martin Koehler, 86–91. Boston: Center for Psychiatric Rehabilitation (Boston University), 1997.

"Housing First." National Alliance to End Homelessness, April 20, 2016. Accessed April 1, 2022. https://endhomelessness.org/resource/housing-first/?msclkid=a2c7065db20011ec8efb938e6962f5e0.

Howell, Alison, and Jijian Voronka. "Introduction: The Politics of Resilience and Recovery in Mental Health Care." *Studies in Social Justice* 6, no. 1 (2012): 1–7.

Huth, Martin. "The Dialectics of Vulnerability: Can We Produce or Exacerbate Vulnerability by Emphasizing It as a Normative Category?" *Philosophy Today* 64, no. 3 (Summer 2020): 557–576.

Jacobson, Nora, and Dianne Greenley. "What Is Recovery? A Conceptual Model and Explication." *Psychiatric Services* 52, no. 4 (April 2001): 482–485.

James, Doris J., and Lauren E. Glaze. "Mental Health Problems of Prison and Jail Inmates." Bureau of Justice Statistics NCJ 213600, September 6, 2006. Accessed August 8, 2022. https://bjs.ojp.gov/library/publications/mental-health-problems-prison-and-jail-inmates.

Janicki-Deverts, Denise, and Sheldon Cohen. "Social Ties and Resilience in Chronic Disease." In *Resilience and Mental Health: Challenges Across the Lifespan*, edited by Steven M. Southwick, Brett T. Litz, Dennis Charney, and Matthew J. Friedman, 76–89. Cambridge: Cambridge University Press, 2011.

Johnson-Kwochka, Annalee, Gary R. Bond, Deborah R. Becker, Robert E. Drake, and Mary Ann Greene. "Prevalence and Quality of Individual Placement and Support (IPS) Supported Employment in the United States." *Administration and Policy in Mental Health and Mental Health Services Research* 44 (2017): 311–319.

Kant, Immanuel. *Grounding for the Metaphysics of Morals*, 3rd edition. Translated by James W. Ellington. Indianapolis, IN: Hackett, 1993.

Karidi, Maria Veroniki, Costas N. Stefanis, Christos Theleritis, Maria Tzedaki, Andreas D. Rabavilas, and Nicholas C. Stefanis. "Perceived Social Stigma, Self-Concept, and Self-Stigmatization of Patient with Schizophrenia." *Comprehensive Psychiatry* 51 (2010): 19–30.

Kavlac, Adam. "The Virtue of Hope." *Ethical Theory and Moral Practice* 18 (2015): 337–354.

Kidd, Ian James. "Can Illness Be Edifying?" *Inquiry* 55, no. 5 (2012): 496–520.

King, Gillian A., Tamzin Cathers, Elizabeth G. Brown, and Elizabeth MacKinnon. "Turning Points: Emotionally Compelling Life Experiences." In *Resilience: Learning from People with Disabilities and the Turning Points in Their Lives*, edited by Gillian A. King, Elizabeth G. Brown, and Linda K. Smith, 31–88. Westport, CT: Praeger, 2003.

Kwong, Jack M. C. "What Is Hope?" *European Journal of Philosophy* 27 (2019): 243–254.

Lear, Jonathan. *Radical Hope: Ethics in the Face of Cultural Devastation*. Cambridge, MA: Harvard University Press, 2006.

Lindh, Inga-Britt, António Barbosa da Silva, Agneta Berg, and Elisabeth Severinsson. "Courage and Nursing Practice: A Theoretical Analysis." *Nursing Ethics* 17, no. 5 (2010): 551–565.

Lotz, Mianna. "Vulnerability and Resilience: A Critical Nexus." *Theoretical Medicine and Bioethics: Philosophy of Medical Research and Practice* 37, no. 1 (February 2016): 45–59.

Luciano, Alison, and Ellen Meara. "Employment Status of People with Mental Illness: National Survey Data from 2009 and 2010." *Psychiatric Services* 65, no. 10 (October 2014): 1201–1209.

Lützén, Kim, and Béatrice Ewalds-Kvist. "Moral Distress and Its Interconnection with Moral Sensitivity and Moral Resilience: Viewed from the Philosophy of Viktor E. Frankl." *Bioethical Inquiry* 10 (2013): 317–324.

Mackenzie, Catriona. "The Importance of Relational Autonomy and Capabilities for an Ethics of Vulnerability." In *Vulnerability: New Essays in Ethics and Feminist Philosophy*, edited by Catriona Mackenzie, Wendy Rogers, and Susan Dodds, 33–59. New York: Oxford University Press, 2014.

Mackenzie, Catriona, Wendy Rogers, and Susan Dodds. "What Is Vulnerability, and Why Does It Matter for Moral Theory?" In *Vulnerability: New Essays in Ethics and Feminist Philosophy*, edited by Catriona Mackenzie, Wendy Rogers, and Susan Dodds, 1–31. New York: Oxford University Press, 2014.

Mancilla, Alejandra. "The Human Right to Subsistence." *Philosophy Compass* 14 (2019): e12618, 1–10. Accessed August 8, 2022. https://compass.onlinelibrary.wiley.com/doi/10.1111/phc3.12618.

Manco, Nicholas, and Sherry Hamby. "A Meta-Analytic Review of Interventions That Promote Meaning in Life." *American Journal of Health Promotion* 35, no. 6 (2021): 866–873.

Marmot, Michael, and Richard G. Wilkinson. *Social Determinants of Health*, 2nd edition. Oxford: Oxford University Press, 2006.

Martin, Adrienne M. *How We Hope: A Moral Psychology*. Princeton, NJ: Princeton University Press, 2014.

Matthews, Steve. "Blaming Agents and Excusing Persons: The Case of DID." *Philosophy, Psychiatry, & Psychology* 10, no. 2 (June 2003): 169–174.

Matthews, Steve, Robyn Dwyer, and Anke Snoek. "Stigma and Self-Stigma in Addiction." *Bioethical Inquiry* 14 (2017): 275–286.

Matthews, Steve, and Jeanette Kennett. "Respecting Agency in Dementia Care: When Should Truthfulness Give Way?" *Journal of Applied Philosophy* 39, no. 1 (February 2022): 117–131.

Mayer, John D., and Michael A. Faber. "Personal Intelligence and Resilience: Recovery in the Shadow of Broken Consciousness." In *Handbook of Adult Resilience*, edited by John W. Reich, Alex J. Zautra, and John Stuart Hall, 94–111. New York: Guilford Press, 2010.

McConnell, Doug, and Anke Snoek. "The Importance of Self-Narration in Recovery from Addiction." *Philosophy, Psychiatry, & Psychology* 25, no. 3 (September 2018): E31–E44.

McGrath, John J. "Variations in the Incidence of Schizophrenia: Data versus Dogma." *Schizophrenia Bulletin* 32, no. 1 (January 2006): 195–197.

McRae, Emily. "Equanimity and Intimacy: A Buddhist-Feminist Approach to the Elimination of Bias." *Sophia* 52 (2013): 447–462.

McRae, Emily. "Equanimity and the Moral Virtue of Open-Mindedness." *American Philosophical Quarterly* 53, no. 1 (January 2016): 97–108.

Meirav, Ariel. "The Nature of Hope." *Ratio* 22 (June 2009): 216–233.

Meyer, Adolf. *Psychobiology*. Springfield, IL: Charles C. Thomas, 1957.

Meyer, Piper S., and Kim T. Mueser. "Resiliency in Individuals with Serious Mental Illness." In *Resilience and Mental Health: Challenges Across the Lifespan*, edited by Steven M. Southwick, Brett T. Litz, Dennis Charney, and Matthew J. Friedman, 276–288. Cambridge: Cambridge University Press, 2011.

Meyers, Diana Tietjens. *Being Yourself: Essays on Identity, Action, and Social Life*. Lanham, MD: Rowman & Littlefield, 2004.

Miller, Sarah Clark. *The Ethics of Need: Agency, Dignity, and Obligation*. New York: Routledge, 2012.

Milona, Michael. "Discovering the Virtue of Hope." *European Journal of Philosophy* 28 (2020): 740–754. doi: 10.1111/ejop.12518.

Montmarquet, James A. *Epistemic Virtue and Doxastic Responsibility*. Lanham, MD: Rowman & Littlefield, 1993.

Moriarty, Jeffrey. "Rawls, Self-Respect, and the Opportunity for Meaningful Work." *Social Theory and Practice* 35, no. 3 (July 2009): 441–459.

Motrico, Emma, Jose A. Salinas-Perez, Maria Luisa Rodero-Cosano, and Sonia Conejo-Cerón. "Editors' Comments on the Special Issue 'Social Determinants of Mental Health.'" *International Journal of Environmental Research and Public Health* 18, no. 3957 (2021): 1–9. https://doi.org/10.3390/ijerph18083957.

Nelson, Hilde Lindemann. *Damaged Identities, Narrative Repair*. Ithaca, NY: Cornell University Press, 2001.

Neuhäuser, Christian. "Structural Injustice and the Distribution of Forward-Looking Responsibility." *Midwest Studies in Philosophy* 38 (2014): 232–251.

Notess, Susan E. "Listening to People: Using Social Psychology to Spotlight an Overlooked Virtue." *Philosophy* 94, no. 370 (October 2019): 621–643.

O'Neill, Onora. "Rights, Obligations, and Needs." In *Necessary Goods: Our Responsibilities to Meet Others' Needs*, edited by Gillian Brock, 95–112. Lanham, MD: Rowman & Littlefield, 1998.

O'Neill, Onora. *Towards Justice and Virtue: A Constructive Account of Practical Reasoning*. Cambridge: Cambridge University Press, 1996.

Ong, Anthony D., C. S. Bergeman, and Sy-Miin Chow. "Positive Emotions as a Basic Building Block of Resilience in Adulthood." In *Handbook of Adult Resilience*, edited by John W. Reich, Alex J. Zautra, and John Stuart Hall, 81–93. New York: Guilford Press, 2010.

Ostafin, Brian D., and Travis Proulx. "Meaning in Life and Resilience to Stressors." *Anxiety, Stress, & Coping* 33, no. 6 (2020): 603–622.

Padgett, Deborah K., Benjamin F. Henwood, and Sam J. Tsemberis. *Housing First: Ending Homelessness, Transforming Systems, and Changing Lives*. Oxford: Oxford University Press, 2016.

Padhy, Meera, and Padiri Ruth Angiel. "Social Support and Emotion Regulation as Predictors of Well-Being." In *Emotion, Well-Being, and Resilience: Theoretical Perspectives and Practical Applications*, edited by Rabindra Kumar Pradhan and Updesh Kumar, 61–76. Palm Bay, FL: Apple Academic Press, 2021.

Palmqvist, Carl-Johan. "Faith and Hope in Situations of Epistemic Uncertainty." *Religious Studies* 55 (2019): 319–335.

Park, Crystal L., and Jeanne M. Slattery. "Resilience Interventions with a Focus on Meaning and Values." In *The Resilience Handbook: Approaches to Stress and Trauma*, edited by Martha Kent, Mary C. Davis, and John W. Reich, 270–282. New York: Routledge, 2014.

Parker, Kelly A. "Introduction: Resilience as a Philosophical Concept." In *Pragmatist and American Philosophical Perspectives on Resilience*, edited by Kelly A. Parker and Heather E. Keith, vii–xviii. Lanham, MD: Lexington Books, 2020.

Parker, Kelly A., and Daniel J. Brunson. "Catastrophe and the Beloved Community: Resources for Resilience in Josiah Royce and Martin Luther King, Jr." In *Pragmatist and American Philosophical Perspectives on Resilience*, edited by Kelly A. Parker and Heather E. Keith, 37–59. Lanham, MD: Lexington Books, 2020.

Pearson, Giles. "Aristotle on the Role of Confidence in Courage." *Ancient Philosophy* 29 (2009): 123–137.

Pembroke, Neil. "Compassionate Care by Clinicians: Insights from the Judeo-Christian and Buddhist Traditions." *Eubios Journal of Asian and International Bioethics* 25, no. 1 (January 2015): 21–24.

Pepper-Smith, Robert, William R. Harvey, and M. Silberfield. "Competency and Practical Judgment." *Theoretical Medicine* 17 (1996): 135–150.

Pereboom, Derk. "Stoic Psychotherapy in Descartes and Spinoza." *Faith and Philosophy: Journal of the Society of Christian Philosophers* 11, no. 4 (1994): 592–625. Article 4. doi: 10.5840/faithphil199411444.

Pettit, Philip. "Hope and Its Place in Mind." *Annals of the American Academy* 592 (March 2004): 152–165. doi: 10.11.77/0002716203261798.

Phillips, Richard. "Curiosity: Care, Virtue and Pleasure in Uncovering the New." *Theory, Culture & Society* 32, no. 3 (2015): 149–161.

Pickard, Hanna. "The Puzzle of Addiction." In *The Routledge Handbook of Philosophy and Science of Addiction*, edited by H. Pickard and S. H. Ahmed, 9–22. London: Routledge, 2018.

Pickard, Hanna. "Responsibility without Blame: Empathy and the Effective Treatment of Personality Disorder." *Philosophy, Psychiatry, & Psychology* 18, no. 3 (September 2011): 209–224.

Pickard, Hanna. "What We're Not Talking about When We Talk about Addiction." *Hastings Center Report* 50, no. 4 (2020): 37–46.

Pienkos, Elizabeth, Anne Giersch, Marie Hansen, Clara Humpston, Simon McCarthy-Jones, Aaron Mishara, Barnaby Nelson, Sohee Park, Andrea Raballo, Rajiv Sharma, Neil Thomas, and Cherise Rosen. "Hallucinations beyond Voices: A Conceptual Review of the Phenomenology of Altered Perception in Psychosis." *Schizophrenia Bulletin* 45, suppl. no. 1 (2019): S72.

Pogge, Thomas. "Are We Violating the Human Rights of the World's Poor?" *Yale Human Rights and Development Journal* 14, no. 2 (2011): 1–33 (Article 1). Accessed February 17, 2022. http://digitalcommons.law.yale.edu/yhrdlj/vol14/iss2/1.

Pogge, Thomas W. *World Poverty and Human Rights: Cosmopolitan Responsibilities and Reforms*, 2nd edition. Cambridge: Polity, 2008.

Potter, Nancy Nyquist. *The Virtue of Defiance and Psychiatric Engagement*. Oxford: Oxford University Press, 2016.

Potter, Nancy Nyquist. "Voice, Silencing, and Listening Well: Socially Located Patients, Oppressive Structures, and an Invitation to Shift the Epistemic Terrain." In *The Bloomsbury Companion to Philosophy of Psychiatry*, edited by Şerife Tekin and Robyn Bluhm, 305–324. London: Bloomsbury Academic, 2019.

Rashed, Mohammed Abouelleil. *Madness and the Demand for Recognition: A Philosophical Inquiry into Identity and Mental Health Activism*. Oxford: Oxford University Press, 2019.

Ratcliff, Kathryn Strother. *The Social Determinants of Health: Looking Upstream.* Cambridge: Polity Press, 2017.
Reich, John W., Alex J. Zautra, and John Stuart Hall. "Preface." In *Handbook of Adult Resilience*, edited by John W. Reich, Alex J. Zautra, and John Stuart Hall, xi-xv. New York: Guilford Press, 2010.
Ren, Songyao. "The Zhuangist Views on Emotions." *Asian Philosophy* 28, no. 1 (2018): 55-67.
Repper, Julie, and Rachel Perkins. *Social Inclusion and Recovery: A Model for Mental Health Practice.* Edinburgh: Ballière Tindall, 2003.
Richards, Donald R., and Thomas L. Steiger. "Value Orientations and Support for Guaranteed Income." *Social Science Quarterly* 102 (2021): 2733-2751.
Rocha, James. "Autonomy within Subservient Careers." *Ethical Theory and Moral Practice* 14 (2011): 313-332.
Roessler, Beate. "Meaningful Work: Arguments from Autonomy." *Journal of Political Philosophy* 20, no. 1 (2012): 71-93.
Rogers, Wendy. "Vulnerability and Bioethics." In *Vulnerability: New Essays in Ethics and Feminist Philosophy*, edited by Catriona Mackenzie, Wendy Rogers, and Susan Dodds, 60-87. New York: Oxford University Press, 2014.
Ross, Lewis. "The Virtue of Curiosity." *Episteme* 17, no. 1 (2020): 105-120.
Rossa-Roccor, Verena, Peter Schmid, and Tilman Steinert. "Victimization of People with Severe Mental Illness outside and within the Mental Health Care System: Results on Prevalence and Risk Factors from a Multicenter Study." *Frontiers in Psychiatry* 11 (2020). https://doi.org/10.3389/fpsyt.2020.563860.
Rudnick, Abraham, ed. *Recovery of People with Mental Illness: Philosophical and Related Perspectives.* Oxford: Oxford University Press, 2012.
Saks, Elyn R. *The Center Cannot Hold: My Journey through Madness.* New York: Hyperion, 2007.
Schrader, Michael, and Michael Levine. "Hope: The Janus Faced Virtue (with Feathers)." *European Journal for Philosophy of Religion* 11, no. 3 (2019): 11-30.
Schwager, Susanne, and Klaus Rothermund. "The Automatic Basis of Resilience: Adaptive Regulation of Affect and Cognition." In *The Resilience Handbook: Approaches to Stress and Trauma*, edited by Martha Kent, Mary C. Davis, and John W. Reich, 55-72. New York: Routledge, 2014.
Scrutton, Anastasia Philippa. "Epistemic Injustice and Mental Illness." In *The Routledge Handbook of Epistemic Injustice*, edited by Ian James Kidd, Jose Medina, and Gaile Pohlhaus Jr., 347-355. London: Routledge, 2017.
Sederer, Lloyd I. "The Social Determinants of Mental Health." *Psychiatric Services* 67, no. 2 (February 2016): 234-235.
Shim, Ruth S., and Michael T. Compton. "Addressing the Social Determinants of Mental Health: If Not Now, When? If Not Us, Who?" *Psychiatric Services* 69, no. 8 (August 2018): 844-846.

Shim, Ruth S., and Michael T. Compton. "The Social Determinants of Mental Health: Psychiatrists' Roles in Addressing Discrimination and Food Insecurity." *Focus* 18, no. 1 (Winter 2020): 25–30.

Shue, Henry. *Basic Rights: Subsistence, Affluence, and U.S. Foreign Policy*. Princeton, NJ: Princeton University Press, 1980.

Simmons, Aaron. "In Defense of the Moral Significance of Empathy." *Ethical Theory and Moral Practice* 17 (2014): 97–111.

Slade, Mike. *Personal Recovery and Mental Illness: A Guide for Mental Health Professionals*. Cambridge: Cambridge University Press, 2009.

Snow, Nancy. "Empathy." *American Philosophical Quarterly* 37, no. 1 (2000): 65–78.

Southwick, Steven M., and Dennis S. Charney. *Resilience: The Science of Mastering Life's Greatest Challenges*, 2nd edition. Cambridge: Cambridge University Press, 2018.

Stansfeld, Stephen A. "Social Support and Social Cohesion." In *Social Determinants of Health*, 2nd edition, edited by Michael Marmot and Richard G. Wilkinson, 148–171. Oxford: Oxford University Press, 2006.

Steele, Ken, and Claire Berman. *The Day the Voices Stopped: A Memoir of Madness and Hope*. New York: Basic Books, 2001.

Steinberg, Darrell, David Mills, and Michael Romero. "When Did Prisons Become Acceptable Mental Health Care Facilities?" Stanford Law School Three Strikes Project, February 9, 2015. Accessed August 8, 2022. https://law.stanford.edu/wp-content/uploads/sites/default/files/publication/863745/doc/slspublic/Report_v12.pdf.

Stichter, Matt. "Ethical Expertise: The Skill Model of Virtue." *Ethical Theory and Moral Practice* 10 (2007): 183–194.

Stichter, Matt. "Virtues as Skills in Virtue Epistemology." *Journal of Philosophical Research* 38 (2013): 333–348.

Strohminger, Nina, and Shaun Nichols. "The Essential Moral Self." *Cognition* 131 (2014): 159–171.

Sullivan, Shannon. *Living Across and Through Skins: Transactional Bodies, Pragmatism, and Feminism*. Bloomington: Indianapolis University Press.

Sullivan, William Patrick. "A Long and Winding Road: The Process of Recovery from Severe Mental Illness." In *Psychological and Social Aspects of Psychiatric Disability*, edited by LeRoy Spaniol, Cheryl Gagne, and Martin Koehler, 14–24. Boston: Center for Psychiatric Rehabilitation (Boston University), 1997.

Swarbrick, Margaret. "A Wellness Approach to Mental Health Recovery." In *Recovery of People with Mental Illness: Philosophical and Related Perspectives*, edited by Abraham Rudnick, 30–38. Oxford: Oxford University Press, 2012.

Syed, Moin, and Kate C. McLean. "Master Narrative Methodology: A Primer for Conducting Structural-Psychological Research." *Cultural Diversity and Ethnic Minority Psychology* 29, no. 1 (2023): 53–63.

Syed, Moin, and Kate C. McLean. "Who Gets to Live the Good Life? Master Narratives, Identity, and Well-Being within a Marginalizing Society." *Journal of Research in Personality* 100 (2022): 1–7, Article 104285.
Taylor, Paul W. *Respect for Nature: A Theory of Environmental Ethics*, 25th Anniversary Edition. Princeton, NJ: Princeton University Press, 1986.
Tekin, Şerife. "The Missing Self in Scientific Psychiatry." *Synthese* 196 (2019): 2197–2215.
Tekin, Şerife. "Patients as Experience-Based Experts in Psychiatry: Insights from the Natural Method." In *The Natural Method: Essays on Mind, Ethics, and Self in Honor of Owen Flanagan*, edited by Eddy Nahmias, Thomas W. Polger, and Wenqing Zhao, 79–97. Cambridge, MA: MIT Press, 2020.
Tekin, Şerife. "Self-Concept through the Diagnostic Looking Glass: Narratives and Mental Disorder." *Philosophical Psychology* 24, no. 3 (June 2011): 357–380.
Tekin, Şerife. "Self-Insight in the Time of Mood Disorders: After the Diagnosis, beyond the Treatment." *Philosophy, Psychiatry & Psychology* 21, no. 2 (June 2014): 139–155.
Thomhave, Kalena. "Money for the People." *The Progressive* (June/July 2021): 41–44.
Thornhill, Hermione, Linda Clare, and Rufus May. "Escape, Enlightenment and Endurance: Narratives of Recovery from Psychosis." *Anthropology & Medicine* 11, no. 2 (August 2004): 181–199.
Throop, William M. "Frugality and Resilience: A Pragmatist Meditation." In *Pragmatist and American Philosophical Perspectives on Resilience*, edited by Kelly A. Parker and Heather E. Keith, 61–80. Lanham, MD: Lexington Books, 2020.
Troy, Allison S., and Iris B. Mauss. "Resilience in the Face of Stress: Emotion Regulation as a Protective Factor." In *Resilience and Mental Health: Challenges Across the Lifespan*, edited by Steven M. Southwick, Brett T. Litz, Dennis Charney, and Matthew J. Friedman, 30–44. Cambridge: Cambridge University Press, 2011.
Turner, Bryan S. *Vulnerability and Human Rights*. University Park: Pennsylvania State University Press, 2006.
United Nations. "International Covenant on Economic, Social and Cultural Rights." United Nations Human Rights Office of the High Commissioner (ratified 1966). Accessed August 8, 2022. https://www.ohchr.org/sites/default/files/Documents/ProfessionalInterest/cescr.pdf.
Walker, Brian, and David Salt. *Resilience Practice: Building Capacity to Absorb Disturbance and Maintain Function*. Washington, DC: Island Press, 2012.
Walker, Margaret Urban. "Hope's Value." In *Moral Repair: Reconstructing Moral Relations after Wrongdoing*, 40–71. Cambridge: Cambridge University Press, 2006.
Weber, Marcela C., Jeffrey M. Pavlacic, Emily A. Gawlik, Stefan E. Schulenberg, and Erin M. Buchanan. "Modeling Resilience, Meaning in Life, Posttrau-

matic Growth, and Disaster Preparedness with Two Samples of Tornado Survivors." *Traumatology* 26, no. 3 (2020): 266–277.

Whitley, Rob, and Benjamin F. Henwood. "Life, Liberty, and the Pursuit of Happiness: Reframing Inequities Experienced by People with Severe Mental Illness." *Psychiatric Rehabilitation Journal* 37, no. 1 (2014): 68–70.

Whitley, Rob, and Robert E. Drake. "Recovery: A Dimensional Approach." *Psychiatric Services* 61, no. 12 (December 2010): 1248–1250.

Widdershoven, A. M. Guy, Andrea Ruissen, Anton J. L. M. van Balkom, and Gerben Meynen. "Competence in Chronic Mental Illness: The Relevance of Practical Wisdom." *Journal of Medical Ethics* 43 (2017): 374–378.

Willoughby, Colleen, Elizabeth G. Brown, Gillian A. King, Jacqueline Specht, and Linda K. Smith. "The Resilient Self—What Helps and What Hinders?" In *Resilience: Learning from People with Disabilities and the Turning Points in Their Lives*, edited by Gillian A. King, Elizabeth G. Brown, and Linda K. Smith, 89–128. Westport, CT: Praeger, 2003.

Woolfrey, Joan. "The Infectiousness of Hope." *Philosophy in the Contemporary World* 22, no. 2 (Fall 2015): 94–103.

Young, Iris M. "Five Faces of Oppression." *Philosophical Forum* 19, no. 6 (1988): 270–290.

Young, Iris Marion. *Responsibility for Justice*. Oxford: Oxford University Press, 2011.

Zagzebski, Linda Trinkaus. *Virtues of the Mind: An Inquiry into the Nature of Virtue and the Ethical Foundations of Knowledge*. Cambridge: Cambridge University Press, 1996.

Zautra, Alex J., John Stuart Hall, and Kate E. Murray. "Resilience: A New Definition of Health for People and Communities." In *Handbook of Adult Resilience*, edited by John W. Reich, Alex J. Zautra, and John Stuart Hall, 3–29. New York: Guilford Press, 2010.

Zolli, Andrew, and Ann Marie Healy. *Resilience: Why Things Bounce Back*. New York: Free Press, 2012.

Index

abuse, 41–42, 138, 141–143, 152, 159
acceptance: as forbearance, 80; by others, 104, 114; definition, 80; of one's situation, 21, 26, 71–74, 80–84, 96, 192, 196
accommodation, 21
action-guiding, 92–93
actions: confluence of, 165; cumulative effects of, 166; positive vs. negative, 137–140
acts of kindness, 190–191
adaptation, 2, 71–72, 74–76, 79–80, 87–88; positive, 21–25, 33, 213. See also adjustment
adjustment, 21–26, 80, 87–88, 192, 196; of expectations, 33, 96. See also adaptation
adversity: and resilience, 26–27; as harm, 49; as obstacles to functioning, 21; in the individual, 28; overcoming, 14–15, 22; reframing, 196; seeking out, 27–28. See also coping, with adversity
agency, 24, 50–55, 210; capacities for, 163–164, 192; constraints, 131, 159–160, 164–166; definition, 18, 61–62; goods for (basic, nonsubtractive, and additive goods), 133–134; justification of duties, 117–118; requirements of (freedom and well-being), 133; social dimension of, 117–118. See also epistemic agency *and* moral agency
alief, 90
assistance: as aid, 5, 107, 117–121, 146; of mental health providers, 107–108. See also duty, of assistance
attitudes, 89–90; and resilience, 80–84, 88–94; definition, 74; positive, 26, 88
author's story, 2–5, 211–212
autonomy, 24, 179; capacities for, 163–164; definition, 18, 61–62; in work, 203; losses of, 54–55
autonomy competency skills. See skills, autonomy competency
autonomy-promoting interventions. See interventions, autonomy-promoting

balance, 15–16
baseline, 15–16, 25
basic needs. See needs, basic
basic rights, 136–137
beliefs, 194–195
belief in possibility, 90
belonging, 104, 187–188, 190–192, 207
beneficence. See duty, of beneficence

255

Index

bouncing back (from adversity), 15, 17

calmness, 80
capacities: basic human, 14–15, 18, 23–26, 28; inner and external, 23–24
capacity, 57–58; to harm, 109–111; to help, 114; to protect, 110–111, 114
care, 108, 117–126; actions, 118–119; dignifying, 123–124. *See also* duty, to protect from harm *and* responsibility
care ethics approach, 117–126
causation of harm, 109–111
certainty, 89
changing a situation, 73–80, 84–88; mentioned, 26, 28, 33, 36, 94, 192
changing the self. *See* self-change
choices in treatment, 107
clinical empathy and compassion, 119
coercion, 41–42, 60, 107, 152; of institutions, 141–142, 146, 149, 157. *See also* restraints
cognitive reappraisal, 195–196, 199–200, 207
colleagues, 107
collective action, 77, 82, 145, 169
comorbidity, 65
compensation. *See* duty, to compensate for harms
competence, 3, 202–203, 205
confidence, 86, 93, 97, 202, 205
conscientiousness, 199
consequentialist approach, 103, 108–117; objections to, 115–116
contingent vulnerability. *See* vulnerability, contingent
contributing to one's own harm, 113–115
contributing to society, 184–186, 201, 204

control: and empowerment, 170; and responsibility, 28–29; and uptake, 179–181; over a situation, 26, 33–34, 75–76, 80, 96; over internals and externals, 82; over medication, 93; over mental illness, 101–102, 114; over mental states, 81–83; over stressors, 22–23; over the self, 23, 30; over what happens to a person, 197
coping: and aid, 113; strategies, 102–104, 119; with adversity, 15–16, 22–27, 33–34, 62, 68, 104–105. *See also* adversity
core function, 18–20, 33
core purpose, 19–20
core self, 88
corporeal vulnerability. *See* vulnerability, corporeal
courage, 84–86, 93, 96–97, 103, 188
creativity, 26, 79–80, 96, 188, 195
credibility, 34, 36, 53, 65–66, 170–172, 177–180
crutch, 99–100
curiosity, 83–84

Deafness, 60–61
deinstitutionalization, 66
deontological approach, 103, 108, 117–126
dependence, 3, 57–58, 113, 117–118, 126; on systems, 59–60, 85, 130, 150, 152. *See also* interdependence
detachment, 81, 83, 174–175
determination, 72–73, 99
dignity, 116, 120, 123–124
discrimination, 142, 146, 149, 159–160
distribution of benefits and burdens, 163–166, 181
distributive justice, 158, 160–161, 163

domination, 53–54, 141–142, 146, 168–169
DSM (*Diagnostic and Statistical Manual*) culture, 49, 198
duties entailed by a right to mental health, 137
duty: conflicts of, 112, 122; imperfect, 112–113, 121–122, 138–140; of assistance, 112, 115, 138–140; of beneficence, 117–118, 121–122, 125; of individuals to get their own needs met, 149–152; perfect, 112–113, 121–122, 138–140; supererogatory, 115; to aid vulnerable individuals, 137–138, 143, 149, 161; to avoid harming, 136–138, 143, 149; to compensate for harms, 137–138, 143, 149; to protect from harm, 108–117, 136–138, 143–144, 149, 161; to reform, 143; universalizability of, 112–113, 117–118, 133, 139–140. *See also* assistance; care; institutional responsibility; listening; responsibility; responsiveness; *and* uptake
duty-bearers, 128

education, 134–137, 139, 143–144, 149, 159–163, 202
embodied subjects, 45–48
emotional support. *See* support, emotional
empathy, 104, 175
employment, 135–144 passim, 149, 156, 159–163, 201, 218–219n8. *See also* work
empowerment, 170–171, 202
encouragement, 101, 106, 115
ends: adopting others', 119–123; helping others pursue, 119–120, 122–123, 179–180, 210; self-chosen, 119–120, 122–125, 134, 164, 173, 179–180
end-setting, 119–120
endurance, 131–132, 192, 194, 196
engagement, 174–176
en-minded subjects, 45–48
epistemic agency, 48, 51–54, 179, 199; losses of, 51–54. *See also* agency *and* moral agency
epistemic agency-promoting interventions. *See* interventions, epistemic-agency-promoting
epistemic community, 34, 95, 113–114, 179, 192
epistemic humility, 81, 89
epistemic injustice, 176
epistemic justice, 172, 233–234n32
epistemic power, 151, 158, 170–171, 178–179
epistemic resources, 119, 151
epistemic subjectivity, 51–54
equanimity, 80–84, 188
equilibrium, 15–16, 24
estrangement, 43
ethics approach to responsibility for mental health, 106–109, 126
expectations, 26, 33, 80–81, 96, 196, 202–203
exploitation, 41–42, 141–142, 146, 155, 165

family members, 43
feedback, 76–77, 176–177
fighting demons, 4–5, 12–14, 99
flexibility, 26, 87–88, 96, 103
flow, 204
fragility of human nature, 46–48, 56
friends, 43, 101, 106, 108, 126
function of a system, 16–17

functioning: enhancement of, 21–22; in life domains, 20–22, 23–25
future-envisioning, 88, 134

giving back, 184–185, 209
goals, 18, 25–28, 33, 78, 134, 179; and meaning, 187, 190, 193–195, 202–204, 207
goal state, 16
good, conception of, 205, 207
good life, liberal framework of, 204–205
gratitude, 190
growth: as sustainability, 16, 22; personal, 11, 24–28, 105–106, 189, 194, 202
guaranteed income, 156, 231n6

harm: additive vs. multiplicative, 142; compounding, 59; environmental, 159–162; hermeneutical, 53; interpersonal, 43, 59; mental, 43; of mental illness, 108; ontological, 145, 147; physical, 43; preventing, 110; risk of, 44, 67, 109; situational, 147–148, 153; social, 42, 145, 165–166; structural, 59, 77. *See also* vulnerability
healthcare, 143, 146, 149, 156, 159–160, 202
health-oriented disposition, 61
hermeneutical harm. *See* harm, hermeneutical
hermeneutical injustice, 53
hermeneutical resources, 54.
homelessness, 40–42, 142, 155–156, 160
hope, 26, 88–94, 195, 197
housing, 139, 143, 146, 149, 159–163, 202
Housing First, 231n4
human rights approach to responsibility for mental health, 133–144, 160, 229–230n19

identity, 16–18, 25, 53, 224n30
identity prejudice credibility deficit, 53
imaginative capacity, 90, 93
impairments, 21, 63
incarceration, 40–41, 65
incompetence, 3
inequalities, 57–58
information, 79
infrastructure, 50, 135
inherent worth, 123
injustice. *See* harm, structural; hermeneutical injustice; institutions, justice of; structural injustice *and* testimonial injustice
insight, 102–103, 198
institutional approach to human rights, 133
institutional approach to meeting mental health needs, 132–133
institutional assets, 147
institutional power, 29–32, 36, 140–144, 163, 167–169, 233n26
institutional responsibility, 29–32, 125–126, 138–149, 233n26; and responsibility for vulnerability, 116; to meet basic needs, 118; to meet the human right to mental health, 132–133, 135–136; to create structural justice, 167–169. *See also* responsibility
institutions: as designed to meet people's needs, 138–141, 145–148, 153, 160–161, 163, 206–207; impoverishment of, 141–142, 146, 153, 168; justice of, 141–143, 146, 153, 156–158, 168; meeting people's needs, 131–133, 144–149; resourcefulness of, 141–143, 146, 153, 168. *See also* responsibility, institutional *and* systems
integrity, 16, 25

intelligibility of reasons, 113
interactional approach to human rights, 133
interdependence, 49–51, 113, 117–118, 126, 142, 145. *See also* dependence
interests, 123
interpersonal approach to meeting mental health needs, 106, 126
interventions: autonomy-promoting, 61–63, 123–124; epistemic-agency-promoting, 61–63; medical, 67; mental illness, 59–63, 67–68, 96; multiplicity of, 64; social, 67; voluntariness of, 130
invulnerability, 113

justice framework of responsibility for mental health, 135
justice in uptake. *See* uptake, justice in

Kantian ethics, 116–118, 125

learning, 24–26; from others, 74, 77, 79, 81–82, 94–96, 103. *See also* skills, learning
liability model of responsibility, 28–29, 169
listening, 76, 119, 151, 158, 171–177; assumptions of, 174; to gain understanding, 172–173, 176; unjust, 175–176
loneliness, 43, 73, 104
losses of mental illness, 96

managing one's situation, 24
marginalization, 136, 141–142, 146
meaning: and purpose, 27, 186–191, 200; finding, 19–20; sources of (belonging, understanding, and doing), 190

meaningful activity, 183–186, 201–207
meaningful life, 1, 5–6, 14, 186, 192, 207
meaning-making, 24, 62, 179; definition, 18–20, 186, 193–194
mental health, 97
mental imaging, 90
mental patients, 66–67
mental states, first-order vs. second-order, 81–84
mental vulnerability. *See* vulnerability, mental
mindfulness, 188, 190, 201
mobilizing support, resources, and/or opportunities, 7, 14, 33–34, 37, 192, 213
moral address, 55
moral agency, 48–49, 51–54, 179; losses of, 54–55. *See also* agency *and* epistemic agency
moral burdens, 115–116
moral community, 95–96, 113–114, 179, 192; participation in, 34, 54, 117, 120
moral identity, 55
moral power, 158
moral response, 55, 112
moral subjectivity, 51–54

narrative construction, 193, 196–201, 207
narratives: illness, 197–198; master, 198; of experience, 49; resourcefulness of, 198–199.
need, 57–58, 131
needs, 117–118, 120–121, 131–133, 136, 145, 201–202; basic, 120–121, 136, 160–162
neglect, 141–143
neoliberal conception of resilience, 30–32
noninterference, 107, 137–138

objections to resilience framework, 27–32. *See also* resilience
ontological vulnerability. *See* vulnerability, ontological
openness, 89, 177, 209
opportunities, 34–35; adequacy of, 146; taking advantage of, 33–35
oppression, 53–54, 136, 141–142, 146, 168–169, 233n29; and pathogenic vulnerability, 60
optimism, 26
options for action, 62
outcomes, 109–111; creating, 75–76, 78

paternalism, 122–123
pathogenic vulnerability. *See* vulnerability, pathogenic
perseverance, 4–5, 11–12, 80–81, 87, 93, 97
personhood, 116, 228n2
physical health problems, 43, 63–66
pluralist approach to responsibility, 103, 108–109
positive adaptation. *See* adaptation, positive
positive psychology movement, 30
possibility, 88–95, 179. *See also* probability
poverty, 42, 58, 73, 159
power: and agency, 163–166; between individuals and institutions, 163–166, 180–181; definition, 75; of the individual, 26, 33, 56–58, 71–78, 96, 210; relations, 158, 170, 180–181; of systems, 147. *See also* institutional power
powerlessness, 61, 64, 72, 80, 156
precarity, 85, 144; of institutions/structure, 46
prejudice, 142–143, 152
Principle of Generic Consistency (PGC), 133

privilege, 35–36, 56–58, 76, 147, 163–166
probability, 89. *See also* possibility
problem-solving, 78–80, 96, 100, 188, 192, 195
professional duties, 119
protection from harm/vulnerability. *See* duty, to protect from harm
psychosis, 3–5, 11–12, 39–40, 73, 97, 100–101
pull-yourself-up-by-your-bootstraps mentality, 99
purposive agency, 133, 150

quality of life, 160

racism, 57, 159
radical hope, 53
reciprocity: of assistance/care, 118, 209; of needs, 120–121
recognition by others, 191–192, 204, 207
recovery, 2, 14, 30, 186–187; definition, 6–7; factors in, 210–211
relationality, 49–51, 142
relationship-building, 172–173
resilience: and recovery, 14; author's definition, 2–3, 14–15, 24, 33, 36; causation, 28–29; definitions and models, 15–27; individualistic, 14, 27–32, 73, 132, 213; traditional models, 14. *See also* objections to resilience framework
resistance, 32–33
resources, 34–35, 147; access to, 131, 157, 164; adequacy of, 146; ecological, 137, 143, 147, 149; epistemic, 34–35, 62–63, 143; existential, 137, 143, 147, 149; human, 147; material, 34–35, 143, 147; mental health, 131, 135–137,

139, 143, 149; social, 143, 147, 188; spiritual, 34–35, 137, 143, 149
responsibility, 28–32; consequentialist, 110–111; for mental health, 99–102; for vulnerability, 109–117; of governments, 144–145, 148. *See also* care; duty, to protect from harm; institutional responsibility
responsiveness, 36, 76–77; duty of, 171, 177–181; to evidence, 90
responsive state, 31, 144–149, 153, 202, 206
restraints, 41, 107, 185. *See also* coercion
right to mental health, 134–136, 150
risk, 22, 26, 52, 55–56
role modeling, 74, 76, 95, 104, 210
role responsibilities, 112

self-advocacy, 72
self-awareness, 11
self-care, 124
self-change, 22–23, 29, 84–88, 94–95; continuous, 16; in response to a situation, 26, 33, 73–75, 79–80
self-chosen ends. *See* ends, self-chosen
self-concept, 49, 191, 197–198, 200
self-efficacy, 93, 195, 198; and meaning, 188, 190; and recognition by others, 191–192, 204; and support, 104; and work/meaningful activity, 202; definition, 75
self-esteem, 134, 156, 184, 195, 198; and meaning, 188, 190; and recognition by others, 191–192, 204; and work/meaningful activity, 202
self-harm, 124
self-knowledge, 11, 102, 151. *See also* self-understanding
self-medication, 65
self-reflection, 105

self-respect, 205
self-sacrifice, 122
self-stigma, 49
self-talk, 12
self-understanding, 49, 190, 198. *See also* self-knowledge
shame, 65
shocks, 16–17
situatedness, 76, 145, 163–166, 168, 170–171; and vulnerability, 45, 55–57
situational vulnerability. *See* vulnerability, situational
skills: and resilience, 78–80; autonomy competency, 78; definition, 74; learning, 78–79; problem-solving, 78–80
social change, 32, 77
social connection model of responsibility, 169
social control, 59
social determinants of mental health, 159–162
social engagement. *See* social interaction
social exclusion, 152
social interaction, 55, 65, 94–96, 103, 106–107, 111–114; and meaning, 187–188, 190–192, 204, 207.
social isolation, 43, 65, 104
social justice, 160, 162–163, 170, 180–181; definition, 156
social justice approach, 158, 161–162
social relationships, 14, 35, 65, 187–188, 191–192, 207
social-structural vulnerability. *See* vulnerability, social-structural
social structures, 48, 50, 59, 156–158, 163–166, 167–168
social support, 34, 188, 191–192, 207; benefits, 103
spectrum right, 134

stability, 15–16, 24
stereotypes, 40–42
stigma, 57, 65–66, 76, 142–143, 152, 239n77
stoicism, 82
stress, 58–59, 104–107, 150, 159, 162, 188–189; and resilience, 19–23, 29
structural causes of resilience, 29, 31
structural harm. *See* harm, structural
structural injustice, 77, 163
structural justice, 161–167, 233n28; approach, 162–167; definition, 158, 163; institutional response to, 167–169
suicidality, 11, 41, 43
support: belonging, 105; emotional, 95, 104–105, 108, 118–119, 136; epistemic, 105; information/appraisal, 105; instrumental, 105
support group, 104
support network, 130–131
suspension of judgment, 82–83
sustainability, 16, 22, 25–26
systems, 59, 129–131, 140, 152, 158, 164; and agency, 50–51, 167–168; resilience of, 16–18. *See also* institutions

technology, 79
testimonial exclusion, 53
testimonial injustice, 53
testimonial justice, 172
testimony, 177–179
total institutions, 168–169
trauma, 41–42, 138, 141, 159

unemployment, 42, 64–66

uptake, 36, 151; justice in, 158, 171, 177–181

values, 194–195
violence, 41–42, 137, 141–143, 149, 152, 157
virtue of the chickadee, 177
virtues, 83–88, 90–91; as skills, 222n7; definition, 74
voice (having a say), 176–177
voices (hearing voices), 12–13, 39–42, 85, 184
vulnerability: as epistemic and moral subjects and agents, 51–55; as openness to being affected, 209; brought about by mental illness, 64–67; compounding, 63–67, 142, 157, 162, 181; contingent, 44–45; corporeal, 45–48; definition, 44; dispositional vs. occurrent, 44; framework, 108; medical, 66–67; mental, 45–48; natural, 63; ontological, 44–57, 144; ontological vs. contingent, 44–45; particular, 55–57; pathogenic, 59–63, 124, 142, 146, 168; situational, 57–67, 157–158, 162, 164, 181; social, 37, 66, 170; social-structural, 48–51; to self, 113–114; universal vs. particular, 45. *See also* harm

willingness, 81–83; to change, 209; to change one's views, 177
willpower, 72–73, 100
work, 183–186, 202–204. *See also* employment